Overcoming Secondary Stress
in Medical and Nursing Practice

Overcoming Secondary Stress

IN MEDICAL AND NURSING PRACTICE

*A Guide to Professional Resilience
and Personal Well-Being*

ROBERT J. WICKS

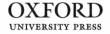

OXFORD
UNIVERSITY PRESS

2006

OXFORD
UNIVERSITY PRESS

Oxford University Press, Inc., publishes works that further
Oxford University's objective of excellence
in research, scholarship, and education.

Oxford   New York
Auckland   Cape Town   Dar es Salaam   Hong Kong   Karachi
Kuala Lumpur   Madrid   Melbourne   Mexico City   Nairobi
New Delhi   Shanghai   Taipei   Toronto

With offices in
Argentina   Austria   Brazil   Chile   Czech Republic   France   Greece
Guatemala   Hungary   Italy   Japan   Poland   Portugal   Singapore
South Korea   Switzerland   Thailand   Turkey   Ukraine   Vietnam

Published by Oxford University Press, Inc.
198 Madison Avenue, New York, New York 10016

www.oup.com

Oxford is a registered trademark of Oxford University Press

Library of Congress Cataloging-in-Publication Data
Wicks, Robert J.
Overcoming secondary stress in medical and nursing practice :
a guide to professional resilience and personal well-being / Robert J. Wicks.
   p. cm.
Includes bibliographical references and index.
ISBN-13 978-0-19-517223-2
ISBN 0-19-517223-X
   1. Physicians—Job stress. 2. Nurses—Job stress. 3. Medical personnel—Job stress.
4. Physicians—Mental health. 5. Nurses—Mental health. 6. Medical personnel—Mental health.
7. Burn out (Psychology)—Prevention. 8. Resilience (Personality trait). 9. Self-care, Health.
10. Stress management. I. Title.
[DNLM: 1. Burnout, Professional—prevention & control. 2. Allied Health Personnel—
psychology. 3. Nurses—psychology. 4. Patient Care—psychology. 5. Physicians—psychology.
WM 172 W6370 2005]
R707.W535 2005
610.69'01'9—dc22   2004026508

9 8 7 6 5 4 3 2 1

Printed in the United States of America
on acid-free paper

Foreword

Denial is one of the best-developed coping reflexes in health care workers, particularly in physicians and nurses. It exists on several levels, and it is provoked by a number of different but related dynamics. Most of us in health care—in the profession of caring for patients—have thought of denial as a self-protective reaction, a shield against the emotional and psychic turmoil of the environment in which we work. And for physicians and nurses, where they work is essentially where they live.

It is a well-worked and commonly described dynamic. It is also oversimplified in its construct and terribly underestimated for its impact on the caregiver's personal well-being and day-to-day effectiveness. There are two levels of denial that deserve particular comment in anticipating the content of this work by Dr. Robert Wicks.

Physicians and nurses are typically trained in hospital settings that afford them exposure to and experience with a remarkable constellation of seriously ill patients. Few of those patients occupy a hospital bed for relatively minor medical problems. In fact, as our health care system has evolved in the United States, the severity of patients' illness in hospital has intensified as everything that is less severe, non–life-threatening, is relegated to nonhospital sites of care. The hospital setting has always been "intense," but over the past 30 years it has become frighteningly, breathtakingly so.

In many hospitals, patients are grouped by clinical discipline—nursing units that consist of all cancer patients, all patients with neurologic diseases, all patients awaiting or having had organ transplantation, and so on. The result is to produce a remarkable concentration of incredibly ill patients whose lives and families are in understandable disarray.

This is the world of physicians and nurses and the reality into which they are immersed from their earliest days of training. It is a world of disease-afflicted lives lined up person-after-person, room-after room in which the physicians and nurses seem to be the only ones spared. Hardly a minute's respite separates one heart-rending, gut-wrenching circumstance from the next. And through this minefield of random misfortune walk the caregivers as if guided by guardian angels, apparently unscathed.

Who among us has not identified with the young leukemia patient who is refractory to treatment and scared to death, or the midcareer professional deeply unresponsive and too young to have had this massive stroke, or the parents trying to absorb into their consciousness the sudden, accidental death of a child? Instead of the afflicted's "Why me?" the caregiver's frightened imponderable becomes "Why not me? What roll of the dice, what act of fate, what divine intervention preserves me from any one of these circumstances?" What makes it possible for physicians and nurses to confront these patients and circumstances day after day with caring and therapeutic resolve and to walk the balance beam between the paralyzing fear of their own mortality and the numbness of emotional disengagement or indifference? And while the hospital environment is the epicenter of personal exposure, the reminders are distributed throughout one's day from office visits with patients to telephone calls with distraught family members. In each encounter, we see ourselves separated from our patients' circumstances by the luck of the draw but believe at a subconscious level that we are somehow protected. It's like wearing a Red Cross arm badge in the battlefield.

There is something self-protective in this construct to be sure. But in fact our effectiveness as physicians and nurses, our value as caregivers resides in the care of the whole person. The ability to do that depends on our ability to empathize with our patients, to see ourselves in our patients. And that, of course, demands that we confront our vulnerability and the statistical likelihood that we, too, will experience the misfortune of illness and its life-changing implications.

To work that through, to reconcile our vulnerability with the need to insulate ourselves from harm, to use that reality to become more effective caregivers requires energy and self-awareness. To fail to do so is a set-up for another level of denial—the inability to appreciate or the refusal to admit the psychological, emotional, and spiritual "wear and tear" of one patient interaction after another. In many ways, patient care is as consumptive for physicians and nurses as illness is for patients. At some point, both parties to the clinical engagement need rest, restoration, and rejuvenation of body and spirit to continue to be effective and useful and, most important, fulfilled. Recognizing this fact, admitting it, and doing something about it require a different level of self-awareness.

It is a fascinating dilemma of patient care that promotes emotional detachment as the platform for rational clinical decision-making but that recognizes identification with patients as the basis for real empathy. The former is almost always achieved only on a conscious, volitional level. The latter is the state to which the good physician or nurse is drawn and strives to achieve. These are complex and traumatizing forces at work.

It is precisely to this circumstance that Robert Wicks applies his keen understanding and insight. Wicks is a clinician whose first-hand knowledge of the patient-caregiver encounter is tell-tale. He understands the environment in which these encounters occur. He understands how physicians and nurses think and, more important, how they feel and articulates both with disarming clarity. Wicks knows his audience and the hazardous world in which they work, and his characterizations of compassion fatigue, burnout, and stress are real-world.

But the description of the problem is not where this book's major contribution lies. Its real value begins with recommendations for assessing the status of one's emotional reserves—or lack thereof—and what to do about it. Wicks holds up a large mirror and walks the observer through a personal inventory using his wisdom and insight as the reader's guide. It is difficult for a physician or nurse to read this book and not feel that the author knows more about you than he should.

This is not a book about self-help. It is a book about self-rediscovery and self-rejuvenation.

Anthony Barbato, M.D.
President, Loyola University Health System

Acknowledgments

As with any project, there are so many people to thank for their suggestions, encouragement, and support. In particular, I would like to thank my colleague Beverly E. Eanes, Ph.D., R.N., for her recommendations about self-care from a nursing perspective; psychiatrist Thomas Cimonetti, M.D., for his reflections on physician stress; Sally Cheston, M.D., for her suggestions on dealing with stress in the radiology/oncology outpatient setting; Anthony Barbato, M.D., for taking out time from his demanding schedule as president of Loyola University Health System in Chicago to write the Foreword to this project; Karyn Felder, my graduate assistant, for aiding in the research and typing; Samuel LaMachia for finding out-of-print books so I could appreciate the long history of writing on the topic of medical/nursing practice and secondary stress; Joseph Ciarrocchi, Ph.D., who as colleague, friend, and department chairperson wholeheartedly supported this project from its inception; James Buckley, Ph.D., Dean of Arts and Sciences, Amanda Thomas, Ph.D., Associate Dean, and the Faculty Development Committee of Loyola College in Maryland for providing me the time and resources to complete the research and write this book; and, of course, my wife, Michaele Barry Wicks, R.N., who made many invaluable suggestions with respect to content, nuance, and editorial presentation of the manuscript—I can't thank her enough for all she did and, more important, who she is.

Permissions

I am grateful for the following permissions to use previously copyrighted material:

Excerpts from *Managing Stress in Emergency Medical Services* by Brian Luke Seaward/American Academy of Orthopaedic Surgeons. Copyright © 2000 Jones and Bartlett Publishers, Sudbury, MA. www.jdpub.com. Used with permission of the publisher.

Excerpts from *Riding the Dragon* by Robert J. Wicks. Copyright © 2003 Sorin Books, an imprint of Ave Maria Press Inc., Notre Dame, IN. www.avemariapress.com. Used with permission of the publisher.

Excerpts from *Simple Changes* by Robert J. Wicks. Copyright © 2000 Thomas More Publishing, an imprint of Ave Maria Press Inc., Notre Dame, IN. www.avemariapress.com. Used with permission of the publisher.

Excerpts from *Touching the Holy* by Robert J. Wicks. Copyright © 1992 by Ave Maria Press, Notre Dame, IN. www.avemariapress.com. Used with permission of the publisher.

Contents

Overcoming Secondary Stress
in Medical and Nursing Practice

Reaching Out . . . Without Being Pulled Down

Remaining Passionate in the Fields of Medicine,
Nursing, and Allied Health—A Guide to Personal
and Professional Well-Being

This book is written for *psychologically healthy* physicians, nurses, and allied health professionals. It is designed to alert them to the sources of secondary stress and provide ways to strengthen their inner lives. In the modern health care setting, knowing this information is not simply desirable; it is essential for one's personal and professional well-being.

If there is an apt proverb for the articulated and unspoken demands many people make of physicians, nurses, and allied health professionals today, it surely must be the Yiddish one: "Sleep faster. . . . We need the pillows!" As physician Simon Brown from the United Kingdom notes in his paper, "The Stresses of Clinical Medicine":

> Perhaps you are thinking that this is the bit that we can all do—
> the "nuts and bolts" clinical doctoring part of medicine. We all
> know how stressful the politics of changing health service has
> been and is likely to continue to be. We all face a daunting
> uphill struggle against piles of paper, the clock, increasingly
> demanding patients, complaints, managing our practices and
> doing more and more for less—just to name but a few of our
> demons. But the clinical medicine is surely the enjoyable bit
> where our training takes over and tells us what to do, even in
> a crisis. After all we are doctors, aren't we?

Of course, the reality of day-to-day clinical practice is different. Despite the training we have already received, there is a disparity between what we achieve and what is expected of us. This gap between supply and demand, both physical and psychological, is an inevitable part of life, let alone work in today's primary care. This is the stuff of stress, the lynchpin of potential unhappiness unless we are able to understand and resolve the difference for ourselves as people, GPs and the profession as a whole. This is an important process. . . . If we get it right, we may just feel contentment in a job well done.[1]

Certainly these comments ring true in different ways for all health care professionals today.

Furthermore, as well as unrealistic expectations on the part of patients and health systems, the stakes are now so high for health care professionals that the potential for developing such psychological problems as emotional blunting on the one hand or extreme affectivity on the other is quite great. Many deny their own emotional needs as a survival mechanism. However, physicians, nurses, and allied health professionals who follow the implicit advice to protect themselves by not allowing themselves to feel too much emotion, sympathy or sadness, run the risk of shutting down entirely in the process.

And so, in their contact with patients, not only may healing professionals contract a physical disease, they are also in an even greater danger of being "infected" psychologically. Secondary stress, *the pressure that results from reaching out to others in need*, is a constant and continuous, reality in medicine, nursing, and allied health. The problem has not disappeared today. It has, in fact, remained a situation to be reckoned with in new ways.

Stress from unfortunate changes in the health care environment, world instability, the internal pressures that result when caring professionals become overwhelmed by frustrations, and the loss of perspective when encountering the inevitable failures of being involved in life and death situations make up only part of a psychologically-combustible mixture. Therefore, to not address this is not only foolish; it is also dangerous to the well-being of a talented, caring, and hitherto emotionally healthy person working in the healing professions—the audience for whom this book is written.

This Book's Framework

Overcoming Secondary Stress in Medical and Nursing Practice is a "one-sitting book" that is designed to distill current clinical papers and research; provide proven guidelines to avoid and/or limit unnecessary distress; strengthen the inner life of physicians, nurses, and allied health personnel; and offer recommendations for further reading on the topic. If nothing else, its goal is to raise awareness that secondary stress is a serious danger. The denial and avoidance of dealing with the immense stress present in modern health care today are amazing. Professionals seem so discouraged at times that they do not even consider—given the culture and their own personal resources—that there are possible practical approaches to deal with environmental and *intra*personal sources of stress in health care settings. Instead, unfortunately, they just march on.

When I had a session with one very competent professional who was starting to manifest early symptoms of chronic secondary stress such as hypersensitivity, increased daily use of alcohol, and sleep disturbance, I asked him how he would characterize his own problem. He said, "I may not be burned out yet." Then, after a brief pause, he smiled slightly and added, "But I think I'm experiencing at least a 'brown out'!" Acknowledging his insight, I asked that given the precarious situation in which he recognized himself, what type of self-care protocol did he design for himself and use to prevent further deterioration of his emotional well-being? In response, after sighing, he said, "I only wish I had the time for something like that!"

Time, of course, is so limited for nurses, physicians, and allied health professionals. More and more I am aware of this even in my own life. Shortly after I received my doctorate from Hahnemann Medical College, a physician who had one of the busiest practices in the area came in for an initial psychological assessment. He was having an affair outside of his marriage. Being a new graduate, I remember carefully formulating a Freudian theoretical diagnosis in my mind. If he were to come in to see me now, though, I must confess that I think my first reaction would be, "Where does he get the time?"

For health professionals, time is especially precious. In response, they need to schedule their priorities and ensure that what is done is accomplished in the most effective way possible. *Overcoming Secondary*

Stress in Medical and Nursing Practice is designed with these realities and practices in mind. This book is a beginning. Nothing more. But a necessary beginning, nonetheless. Without a clear awareness of the challenges of professional health care and the simple, yet powerful, ways to remain a passionate, psychologically healthy nurse, physician, or allied health professional and appreciate the need to strengthen one's "inner life," one's career may become derailed and one's personal life unduly suffer.

This book, as a whole, is presented in a way that provides information that will quickly enable a sufficient appreciation of the essential elements of the problem. Most of these will be obvious; some may prove quite surprising. Following this, guidelines for the development of a personally designed self-care protocol will be provided, as well as information on maintaining perspective and increasing self-knowledge as a way of learning and benefiting from, rather than just being pulled down by, the stressful encounters that will certainly arise.

A major portion of the research and clinical papers over the past 10 years and related books released in the past 25 years have been reviewed in the preparation of this volume. The bibliography in this volume is one of the most extensive and current lists that can be found in any book on this topic published to date. This invaluable material provides grounding for my almost 30 years of clinical experience with physicians, nurses, and allied health professionals. Beyond what is written in the four chapters and epilogue, these sources—especially the ones particularly emphasized after each chapter—also provide wonderful follow-up reading for those wishing to do so.

As was noted, the brevity of the book is also intentional, because of my awareness of the time constraints present. The goal then is to provide a concise, practical (I hope engaging) authored book that incorporates current clinical work and research in a way that avoids the pitfalls of unevenly edited works. It is also designed to be more immediately useful than much earlier oft times out-of-print books. Finally, it is set up to be more focused than longer, wider-ranging volumes that cover ground that is very useful (which can provide added resources for those desiring to read further) yet is unnecessary in a primer on the topic for busy practitioners, as this book is designed to be.

In my experience, too often volumes on the topic of secondary stress and medical/nursing practice have tried to accomplish too much. They simultaneously addressed audiences beyond the physicians, nurses, and allied health professionals themselves. For instance, such works might also contain sound information for therapists treating impaired health professionals and for persons involved in hospital administration and planning. These volumes often devoted a great deal of time to the *already* impaired professional. Although this information is quite valuable, it is not immediately pertinent for our purposes here because this clinical guide is written primarily for those *psychologically healthy* physicians, nurses, or allied health professionals who want to avoid and limit as much as is possible the secondary stress in their own lives and at the same time remain passionate about their work.

Persons in the medical arena realize that "for every poisoned worker there are a dozen with sub-clinical toxicity."[2] Using this as a metaphor for the problem of secondary stress, we need to also realize that for every case of serious impairment, there are many nurses, physicians, and allied health professionals who are starting to manifest some of the symptoms of chronic or acute secondary stress but may not even realize it until well after the fact. This can be appreciated in the following words of Cheryl L. Mee, the editor-in-chief of *Nursing2002*:

> There's one time in my career I look back on with regret. As a young nurse, I frequently worked overtime in high-acuity critical care units. . . . One of the hospitals where I worked was in the city. Most of the patients were poor, with multiple health problems.
>
> Many of them had a poor prognosis and were kept alive with machines—so many in fact that tending to the technology left little time to connect with the humans attached to it. I started to feel like a machine myself. Working too many hours at a breakneck pace in a difficult setting was taking its toll.
>
> Because I worked as a float nurse in various units, I hadn't bonded with the other nurses. But as I began to doubt my career choice, I found myself confiding in one of them. I confessed that the technology and the lack of interaction with my patients made me feel like a robot and I couldn't see how I was helping anyone. She seemed horrified and couldn't relate to my feelings at all. Alienated and ashamed, I thought I was a terrible nurse and wanted to quit. Now I realize that I was a victim of burnout.[3]

Given this, I believe a clinically sound book can be proactive in helping nurses, physicians, allied health professionals, and everyone in a field in which significant impairment is a constant possibility when care is not taken to understand, prevent, and carefully confront the personal and systemic sources of secondary stress.

As was mentioned earlier, the most insidious danger to nurses, physicians, and allied health professionals is *denial*. Fortunately, this factor atrophies of its own accord once we accept the following simple reality:

> The seeds of secondary stress and the seeds of true passionate involvement in the fields of medicine, nursing, and allied health are actually the *same* seeds.

The question is not *whether* stress will appear and take a toll on those working in health care; it is to what extent do professionals take essential steps to appreciate, minimize, and learn from this stress to continue—and even deepen—their roles as helpers and healers. Understanding stress unique to health care work and developing a personal self-care protocol can help immeasurably in this regard, and that is what *Overcoming Secondary Stress in Medical and Nursing Practice* is designed to encourage.

To accomplish this, the opening chapter ("Tacking on Dangerous Psychological Waters") concerns chronic secondary stress (often referred to as "burnout" or "compassion fatigue") and its acute counterpart, "vicarious posttraumatic stress." It also begins to address the role that the toxic parts of the health care system play in exacerbating personal stress.

Chapter Two ("Riding the Dragon") distills essential information on approaches to increasing self-awareness—again, in a user-friendly format designed to save time for the busy physician, nurse, and allied health professional by summarizing material on increasing emotional resilience that is normally available only in psychology and psychiatry volumes. Included here is also a specially designed "Medical/Nursing Professional Secondary Stress Self-Awareness Questionnaire," which is introduced to allow readers to create their own profile with respect to their vulnerability and strength and the pressures of life in this demanding field. By using it alone, with a mentor, or in a small group, it can aid in providing information that will improve self-awareness and stress prevention in the medical setting.

Chapter Three ("Drawing from the Well of Wisdom") is a unique section—not presently covered as extensively in other volumes for physicians, nurses, and allied health professionals—on how core spiritual wisdom from a world-religion perspective—and the applied psychology that evolves from this—can be used in one's life as a way of keeping perspective, balance, and a renewed sense of meaning. This material distills the core of some of the writing I have done on the topic during the past 20 years and is provided here with an eye to what would be practical and essential for medical/nursing professionals—whether they are religious or not—to consider, given their intense work, rich personal lives, and important sense of mission.

Chapter Four ("The Simple Care of a Hopeful Heart") builds on and evolves from the previous three chapters. It presents practical guidelines on developing a personally designed self-care protocol to decrease vulnerability to the natural pressures of being a professional in the health care setting. As in the preceding chapters, there are exercises that can be completed to improve self-awareness as a systematic way to improve one's approach to self-care and to strengthening one's inner life.

Finally, as the brief epilogue's title ("Passionate Journeys") indicates, this book is also about maintaining and increasing the passion one originally had for being a professional in the healing arts. Everything that initially attracted people to this fascinating, meaningful, and rewarding profession is still present in some form. However, care must be taken to preserve and enhance a sense of personal and professional well-being and perspective so this outlook is not lost. No one will do this for you. Yet, with a little knowledge and steady effort, appreciation of the wonders of medicine need never be lost for long by the health care professional who truly cares about the physical and emotional welfare of others. Instead, by using knowledge and humility (the two key elements of wisdom) when faced with the stress of the work, one's passion and commitment can actually deepen and mature. The goal of this brief work is based squarely on this belief and hope.

A final caution: There is a great deal of internal and environmental pressure to deny, distort, or avoid the sources of stress. One simple example: A psychiatrist, who works with seniors in medical school regarding their needs and self-care, shared with me that the fear of appearing to be vulnerable that was part of previous dysfunctional styles in physicians is still present. When he asked how many of them were afraid while making rounds in the hospital, not one hand went up. It is almost as if the old dictum for physicians—See one, do one, teach one—carries with it an implicit message: "It's all in the procedure. As far as vulnerability or burnout is concerned—well, that is for social workers!"

Yet, when there is honesty and humility, natural fears and hesitations and the stress they bring with them are recognized as part and parcel of caring for people's lives. It may appear in different forms at different times. In the beginning, the medical field attracts people who tend to be autonomous, leaders, the brightest, and maybe in some cases, even arrogant. Then the reference group changes—there is a whole lecture hall full of bright talented individuals. One no longer stands out.

At another point, the seriousness of the impact of what is being done may dawn. It may occur when the first incision is made as the scalpel is drawn through the top layer of skin, medication is prescribed or administered, a treatment is given, or an emergency requires action.

Maybe the source of the stress is the financial worries, the fear of a malpractice suit (deserved or not), or the fear of political intrusion; an example would be guidelines imposed by the U.S. Food and Drug Administration that prevent the seemingly appropriate trial use of psychotropic medications normally not used with adolescents in the United States but already having fairly impressive trial results in the United Kingdom.

Possibly it is the interpersonal pressures caused by managing one's office staff, stress in one's marriage, a disruptive physician/nurse/aide on one's unit, the absence of expected status/financial reward for being in the health field, or a surprisingly strong grief response to a patient, such as a young cancer patient who dies suddenly. The list seems endless.

Adding to all of these problems are the offered solutions that in themselves seem unrealistic. Stress prevention courses are offered in most medical/nursing/allied health schools and continuing education programs. However, when a list of the problems that health care providers must face is presented and reviewed, the oft heard "back of the room" response by those attending is, "Yes, I knew that all along. So what. There's nothing you can do about it. It is part of the territory." Then, when a long list of stress-reducers is subsequently offered, unconsciously the response to that may also be to put these recommendations in a "mental draw" marked "Nice if I had the time or energy but totally unrealistic given the myriad demands of my schedule."

And, to some extent, this may well be true. After all, to be honest, who has the time for half of what is suggested in these workshops? Even pondering some of these recommended time-consuming stress-reduction steps may seem stressful! On the other hand, denying the dangers posed by secondary stress and resisting a reasonable process of self-knowledge and self-care under the guise that it too is impractical must be circumvented. Given this distinction, the premise of this book is tied to a significantly different question than was just posed: "Who in their right mind would not take out the time to ponder the *essentials* of self-knowledge, self care, and secondary stress?"

The simple reality is that how you answer this question after reading and working with this book (through testing the steps suggested) affects the overall quality of your professional and personal life. Setting aside or denying simple steps designed to increase self-care/knowledge and awareness of secondary stress is not realistic. Given all that health professionals must face, to do so would be an act of dangerous denial. Moreover, it would be quite foolish.

With the bit of guidance offered in this brief book, paradoxically it can take so little to change so much in terms of the outcome of how you live out your life in this wonderful yet challenging profession. The important thing is to understand, plan, act, and review your steps alone or with others. Accordingly, the goal of this book is to structure this process in the most efficient way possible and to intrigue you so that you recognize the challenges, begin acting to strengthen your inner life, and eventually read further in the recommended books and articles. Doing this not only is beneficial to you but also will have a positive impact on the treatment team, of which you are a part; on your patients; and on those with whom you interact in your personal life. The positive ripples are as or more significant for medical/nursing professionals than in any other allied profession for it can, in the end, be a matter of life or death, and you know as well as I do that this is no exaggeration.

Objectives of the Introduction

- Understand the meaning and effects of "secondary stress"
- Recognize that denial and avoidance of considering the role of stress in modern health care is a significant danger to the psychological well-being of physicians, nurses, and allied health professionals
- Appreciate that no matter how healthy you are, stress is part and parcel of involvement in medicine, nursing, and allied

health. (The seeds of secondary stress in the health care field and the seeds of passion about medicine and nursing are actually the *same* seeds.)

- Know that four important elements in preventing, limiting, and learning from the occurrences of secondary stress are (1) awareness of the dangers of the acute and chronic versions of it and being in tune with the toxic environmental factors that are common in health care; (2) appreciating the necessity of developing one's self-care protocol; (3) knowing ways to strengthen one's inner life; and (4) seeing the value of taking the steps necessary to increase self-knowledge as a way of enhancing personal and professional well-being.

Additional Books to Consider

(This section follows each chapter. The full citations for the books listed can be found in the Bibliography.)

The Handbook of Physician Health, edited by Goldman, Myers, and Dickstein, is the best overview of the issues involved in the well-being of physicians; much of this material will also be applicable to the nursing and allied health professional. Chapters that I found of particular relevance to the topic of secondary stress are "Physician temperament, psychology and stress" (Notman); "Physician and intimate relationships" (Myers); "Disruptive behaviors, personality problems, and boundary violations" (Gendel); and "Medical students and residents: Issues and needs" (Dickstein).

From the nursing perspective, one of the most recent books is Sandra Thomas' *Transforming Nurses' Stress and Anger* (Second Edition). It is the best book available on the toll that modern health care can take on nurses, and it is the most positively prescriptive one in terms of how current challenges can be faced. There are many fine books on stress and nursing that were published in the 1980s and still have great relevance today. They are cited at the end of Chapter One and in "Bibliography."

The Academy of Orthopaedic Surgeons sponsored Brian Seward's very helpful work for emergency medical services personnel entitled *Managing Stress in Emergency Medical Services*. This basic treatment of the topic would be helpful for anyone in health care.

Notes

1. S. Brown, "The Stresses of Clinical Medicine," in D. Haslam (Ed.), *Not Another Guide to Stress in General Practice!*, second edition (Oxford: Radcliffe Medical Press, 2000), 52.

2. D. Block, "Foreword," in C. D. Scott and J. Hawk (Eds.), *Heal Thyself: The Health of Healthcare Professionals* (New York: Brunner Mazel Publishers, 1986), ix.

3. C. Mee, "Battling Burnout," *Nursing2002* 32 (2002), 8.

ONE

Tacking on Dangerous Psychological Waters

*Appreciating the Factors Involved in Chronic
and Acute Secondary Stress*

Secondary stress represents the stress caused by the pressures placed on professionals who care for others in need. To understand its various causes, symptoms, and methods of prevention and ways to limit it, it is helpful to break down secondary stress into three components:

- Chronic secondary stress—also known as "burnout" and "compassion fatigue"
- Acute secondary stress—sometimes referred to as "vicarious posttraumatic stress disorder (PTSD)"
- Unique unhealthy aspects of the medical health care culture

With an appreciation of these three components, we begin to realize the many systemic stresses in medicine and nursing that must be faced. We also realize that there are inner resources and personal growing edges that will come to the forefront in the process of meeting them.

There is no getting around the obstacles. In many cases, it is also not possible to remove them. Instead, facing them is like tacking through rough waters. In his book *First You Have to Row a Little Boat*, Richard Bode describes this approach quite well:

> To tack a boat, to sail a zigzag course, is not to deny our destination or our destiny—despite how it may appear to those who never dare to take the tiller in their hand. Just the oppo-

site: It's to recognize the obstacles that stand between ourselves and where we want to go, and then to maneuver with patience and fortitude, making the most of each leg of our journey, until we reach our landfall.[1]

To my mind, "tacking" is an ideal metaphor for the way physicians, nurses, and allied health personnel must face pressures in general, and chronic secondary stress in particular, in the field of health care today. To ignore what must be faced or to simply seek to take everything head on may be disastrous both personally and professionally. On the other hand, knowledge and maturity help us to psychologically tack the stressful waters that must be encountered at times so we can make the most of all that we face as caregivers.

Chronic Secondary Stress

Russian playwright Anton Chekhov once proclaimed, "Any idiot can face a crisis—it's this day-to-day living that wears you out." According to a University of Washington study, three of four medical residents are suffering from what is commonly referred to as "burnout."[2] While this may not significantly affect patient care, according to a study by Linda Hawes Clever reported in the *Annals of Internal Medicine*, slightly more than half the residents experiencing chronic secondary stress reported at least one "suboptimal" patient care practice during the month as opposed to the 20% who were not reportedly suffering from burnout.

The poor practice included making treatment or medication errors that were "not due to a lack of knowledge or inexperience," failing to fully discuss treatment options and answer patients' questions, and discharging patients "because the team was too busy." As Clever, a physician from California Pacific Medical Center in San Francisco, also aptly notes in an editorial that accompanies this study, "We cannot relieve the suffering of others if we, ourselves, are suffering."[3] Such unfortunate suffering can occur slowly, quietly, almost imperceptibly.

The psychiatrist in the novel *The Case of Lucy Bending* laments in a way that rings all too true for all medical and nursing professionals in real life:

Most laymen, he supposed, believed psychiatrists fell apart under the weight of other people's problems. Dr. Theodore

Levin had another theory. He feared that a psychiatrist's life force gradually leaked out. It was expended on sympathy, understanding, and the obsessive need to heal and help create whole lives. Other people's lives. But always from the outside. Always the observer. Then one day he would wake up and discover that he himself was empty, drained.[4]

An Insidious Unnecessarily Unhealthy Culture

Communications theorist Marshall McLuhan once posed the following question: "If the temperature of the bath rises one degree every ten minutes, how will the bather know when to scream?"[5] In no setting is this question a more apt one to consider than in health care settings that reinforce the unhealthy lifestyles of their staffs—oft times under the guise of good patient care. Emily Smythe in her book *Surviving Nursing* recognizes this and points it out by noting a series of myths that pervade the profession: "Myths about nurses, as we know, come from stereotypes. They also come from society's, nursing educators', and nurses' *wishes* for what nurses *should* be . . . [One myth is:] *A "good" nurse cares for all patients equally and is concerned about people all of the time.* This is an expectation. The "should" is implicit. A good nurse *should* care. Yet nurses, even good nurses, soon realize that it is impossible to care for all people equally, and it is also impossible to care for people adequately, given today's workload and system constraints. It is impossible for a nurse to care all the time, yet the expectation persists, not only externally but internally, and many nurses who do not or cannot care enough feel guilty, stressed, or burned out."[6]

During the Grand Rounds I have led on the topic of medical practice and secondary stress, I discussed the important balance that has to be met. On the one hand, contemporary medicine is intense. Long hours, poor staffing, life and death decisions, necessary paperwork, and relationships with staff and patients all take their toll. On the other hand, there are elements in health care that have crept quietly into the culture that can be changed or handled individually and systemically in ways that lessen unnecessary stress. If this is not done, the problem just perpetuates itself. As one practicing physician who was interviewed for a study on residents in family medicine said about the carryover of the time pressures he experienced in training, "You may be able to get out of the residency, but it's real hard to get the residency out of you." Workaholism, sleep deprivation, and other stresses of training are often left unexamined and taken as part and parcel of the medical scene. Careful examination of this situation though leads to other, more hopeful conclusions than this.

Eanes also makes the following three points to demonstrate the nuances to the reality of stress when speaking about the nursing field today:

> In addition to the nursing shortage in general, there is a profound shortage in the long-term workforce which includes many nurses in direct care and supervisory roles. As we all know, the aging segment of the population is expanding rapidly, which will necessitate even more nurses. As Diana Mason notes: "Older adults account for almost half of all days of hospitalization, 69% of home care, and 83% of skilled nursing facility care" (*American Journal of Nursing*, August 2004, 11.)
>
> Through the Red Cross, more than 40,000 nurses (volunteer or paid) are members of DATs (disaster action teams) used for natural and manmade disasters. Now, since 9/11 and with further terrorist threats nurses have been asked to train and volunteer to assist in emergency (Homeland Security) situations. Over their professional careers, nurses have volunteered much of their time due to their compassionate natures and a desire to improve the community locally, nationally, and for some nurses even the wider world community.
>
> Research has shown that due to increased demands upon nurses, not only are patients put at risk, but so are the nurses themselves, both physically and emotionally. Nurses will need to take care of themselves not only emotionally, but also to avoid preventable conditions due to smoking obesity, hypertension, etc. Of course this can be a vicious cycle due to stress.[7]

These points and a myriad of other factors make it imperative that we have a greater understanding of chronic secondary stress (burnout, compassion fatigue) if self-understanding and care are to be based on sound awareness of the challenges and dangers present in health care.

Definition and Causes of Burnout

Edelwich and Brodsky, in one of the first academic book-length treatments of the topic of burnout, defined it as a "progressive loss of idealism, energy, and purpose experienced by people in the helping professions."[8] Freudenberger, who coined the term "burnout," described it as "a depletion or exhaustion of a person's mental and physical resources attributed to his or her prolonged, yet unsuccessful striving toward unrealistic expectations, internally or externally derived."[9]

Since Freudenberger introduced this term, the concept of burnout has been questioned as to its necessity because the same symptoms and signs are seen in other disorders (depression, anxiety). So, when referring to burnout and the interventions needed to prevent or limit it, some professionals feel it is confusing the issue unnecessarily. However, many in the field, including myself, feel that the term is still quite helpful. If for nothing else, it makes it legitimate for persons in the healing and helping professions to experience stress, anxiety, depression, and other negative feelings. Moreover, it provides an integrated way to look at the emotional stress that health care workers experience in their work.

The causes for burnout are legion. As Pfifferling helps us to appreciate, trying to pin down one source of impairment that health care professionals need to be aware of is futile. "As with diseases or conditions that do not have a single cause, there are multiple suggestions as to the origin, contributing factors, and types of susceptible hosts."[10]

In an article on the topic of burnout, psychiatrist James Gill wryly notes that "helping people can be extremely hazardous to your physical and mental health."[11] He goes on to indicate who are good candidates for burnout:

Judging from the research done in recent years, along with clinical experience, it appears that those who fall into the following categories are generally the most vulnerable: (1) those who work exclusively with distressed persons; (2) those who work intensively with demanding people who feel entitled to assistance in solving their . . . problems; (3) those who are charged with the responsibility for too many individuals; (4) those who feel strongly motivated to work with people but who are prevented from doing so by too many administrative paperwork tasks; (5) those who have an inordinate need to save people from their undesirable situations but find the task impossible; (6) those who are very perfectionistic and thereby invite failure; (7) those who feel guilty about their own human needs (which, if met, would enable them to serve others with stamina, endurance and emotional equanimity); (8) those who are too idealistic in their aims; (9) those whose personality is such that they need to champion underdogs; (10) those who cannot tolerate variety, novelty, or diversion in their work life; and (11) those who lack criteria for measuring the success of their undertakings but who experience an intense need to know that they are doing a good job.

Most researchers and authors on the topic of burnout have developed their own tailored list (Table 1-1) of the causes of burnout, but "there is much overlap, and all seem to point to the problem as being a *lack* that produces frustration. It can be a deficiency—the lack of education, opportunity, free time, ability, chance to ventilate, institutional power, variety, meaningful tasks, criteria to measure impact, coping mechanisms, staff harmony, professional and personal recognition, insight into one's motivations, balance in one's schedule, and emotional distance from the client population. . . . And because these factors are present to some degree in every human services setting, the potential for burnout is always present."[12]

Consequently, every healing professional is in danger of impairment in some way *to some extent*. Yet, care is provided in most settings only to those professionals who are so seriously impaired as to be required by their state boards to seek out help. Although an impaired physician/nursing program is essential, as in the case of physical problems, prevention or early treatment is obviously a preferable step to later intervention. However, as a clinical report in the *Annals of Internal Medicine* notes, "Self care is not a part of the physician's professional training and typically is low on a physician's list of priorities. 'Physicians deal with [other people's] problems all day, but they're the least likely to raise their own personal problems. They don't easily admit that they're under stress,' remarked [neurologist T. Jock] Murray. Approximately one third of physicians do not have a doctor according to a recent study that examined graduates of the Johns Hopkins School of Medicine."[13]

Two of the most knowledgeable clinicians aware of the challenges of being a physician today are Wayne and Mary Sotile. They have

Table 1-1 Causes of Burnout

1. Inadequate quiet time—physical rest, cultural diversion, further education, and personal psychological replenishment
2. Vague criteria for success and/or inadequate positive feedback on efforts made
3. Guilt over failures and over taking out time to nurture oneself properly to deal with one's own legitimate needs
4. Unrealistic ideals that are threatening rather than generally motivating
5. Inability to deal with anger or other interpersonal tensions
6. Extreme need to be liked by others, prompting unrealistic involvement with others
7. Neglect of emotional, physical, and spiritual needs
8. Poor community life and/or unrealistic expectations and needs surrounding the support and love of others for us
9. Working with people (peers, superiors, those coming for help) who have burnout
10. Extreme powerlessness to effect needed change or being overwhelmed by paperwork and administrative tasks
11. Serious lack of appreciation by our superiors, colleagues, or those whom we are trying to serve
12. Sexism, ageism, racism, or other prejudice experienced directly in our lives and work
13. High conflict in the family, home, work, or living environment
14. Serious lack of charity among those with whom we must live or work
15. Extreme change during times in life when maturational crises and adjustments are also occurring (e.g., a 48-year-old physician who is being asked to work with patients diagnosed with cancer at a time when she has just been diagnosed with cancer herself)
16. Seeing money wasted on projects that seem to have no relation to helping people or improving the health care system
17. Not having the freedom or power to deal with or absent oneself from regularly occurring stressful events
18. Failure to curb one's immature reasons for helping others and to develop more mature ones in the process.
19. The "savior complex"—an inability to recognize what we can and cannot do in helping others in need
20. Overstimulation or isolation and alienation

worked as consultants to more than 400 medical organizations. In addition, they have specialized in the area of marriage and family counseling involving physicians.[14]

In their latest book on effective emotional management for physicians and their medical organizations, one of their unique contributions is to bring together some of the research on physician stress under the theme of "betrayal." To use their wording, "Remember: Stress that is highly demanding but also meaningful and controllable is healthy stress, not the sort that promotes burnout. Our counseling and consulting experience suggest that what *really* stresses physicians is feeling betrayed, or double-crossed."[15]

To give a sense of what they mean by this, they quote one of the physicians from a Canadian survey by Sullivan and Burke that they found especially useful:

> I believe that most physicians unconsciously contracted with society to pursue their profession to the utmost of their ability and energy, to keep up their skills and do whatever was needed to promote patient care. In return, we expected respect, the equipment to do the job and freedom from financial anxieties. All 3 of these expectations have been abrogated, yet we continue to fulfill our side of the contract in confusion, disbelief and a sense of betrayal.[16]

They go on to point out that what they term "relationship stress" is a key element in physician burnout. Sources for this, they suggest, center around five areas: "loss of autonomy; changes in patient-physician relationship; work-family conflicts; conflicts with peers, staff, and administrators; and a lack of collegiality particularly in the wake of having made a mistake."

The fact that they have chosen to emphasize these areas certainly seems more than appropriate—especially in terms of loss of autonomy and conflict within their relationships at work and at home. With respect to *loss of autonomy*, it is when persons perceive they have an impact on their work environment (whether in reality they do or do not) that they are less apt to experience the degree of stress they would have if they had no control at all. With the advent of large health maintenance organizations and new insurer norms, physicians in particular have felt a dramatic decrease in control. When the impact of this starts to psychologically "infect" a medical organization, it can set the stage for group burnout, because negativity is so emotionally contagious.

Changes in patient-physician relationships and *conflicts with peers, staff, and administration* are the other two areas on which the Sotiles focus that I find particularly helpful to recognize. In relationships with patients, it is easy for health care professionals to identify with the stress that can arise from interactions with persons who relate in a difficult manner.

There are classic styles that fit into this category (e.g., passive aggressive, overtly hostile, demanding especially with respect to time, etc.). In response to this, one of my colleagues uses humor as one of his coping devices. Recently, he quipped: "I really think there are only five difficult patients in the world and they just move from hospital to hospital."

Sometimes a patient becomes difficult to deal with for a myriad of reasons (e.g., the health care professional is exhausted from being on call all night or completing a 12-hour shift), and this inadvertently exacerbates the situation. In one observation of interactions in a pediatric emergency department, I noted the different styles of workers and how it affected one patient. A 30-year-old woman brought in her youngest child, a 1½-year-old, who was having respiratory problems and a rising fever. When she first brought the child in at midnight, both the physician (who was struggling with English, because he was from the western part of Africa) and the nurse listened carefully to the problem, explained possible causes, and suggested several approaches. Once the approach was agreed on, treatment was careful, kind, and swift. The mother of the patient reported to me her great satisfaction with the treatment provided for her child and the information given to her.

When the woman had to revisit the same emergency department the next morning to clarify one of the forms of treatment and to request assistance with it, she encountered three physicians and a nurse when she entered the unit. She noted that not one of them stood to greet her; instead, they remained sitting with stethoscopes hanging around their neck. The power differential was obvious. As the mother explained her needs, they seemed confused and impervious as to how to meet them. As the woman became more fearful about whether her needs would be met, one of the physicians became more strident as to what she should do. When the woman expressed anger, rather than letting her ventilate and express understanding as to how she felt, the physician kept repeating to the child's mother, "*You* are not listening. *You* are not listening!" I was very surprised that the physician in question did not realize that in fact the patient was not the only one having a problem listening. The physician was not listening to the emotions covering the fear this mother was feeling about her child. The situation could have been deflated before it became a stressful situation for both the patient and the physician. The overall lesson is that there is enough unavoidable stress in the health care setting without communicating to both patients and colleagues in a way that unnecessarily increases stress. After

Table 1-2 Conflicts with Peers, Staff, and Administrators

Peer Conflict

Schedules and calendars
Approaches to patient management
Sharing workload
Clinic or laboratory space
Management of budget for a group/unit
Balancing patient care, teaching, and research
Authorship disputes
Failure to deal with their low performers

Conflict with People Whom Physicians Supervise

Conflict among supervisees that compromises work
Expectations for performance
Dealing with the low performer
Workloads and schedules
Inappropriate personal relationships at work
Volume and quality of work
Interactions with supervisor
Unwillingness to change practice or behavior
Supervision outside the hierarchy

Conflict with Authority Figures

Disagreement about values
Lack of consistency in their actions
Micromanagement
Unfair treatment
Discrimination
Salary negotiations
Broken promises
Clinical and other workload
Ethical dilemmas

Source: W. M. Sotile and M. O. Sotile, *The Resilient Physician* (Chicago: American Medical Association, 2002)—summarized from study conducted by C. A. Aschenbrener and C. T. Siders, "Managing Low-to-Mid Intensity Conflict in the Health Care Setting," *The Physician Executive* 25 (1999): 44-50.

all, when the patients or, as in the case of pediatric and geriatric cases, their families have increased stress due to poor physician/nurse-patient communications, who ultimately is the recipient of the patient's ire? It is the caregiver. However, it is not easy for any of us in health care to have a sufficiently sound level of self-awareness to pick up on this on every occasion. As W. H. Auden aptly noted, "conscious insensitivity is a self-contradiction."[17] (See the discussion in Chapter 2 on approaches to self-awareness.)

In terms of conflict with peers, staff, and administrators, Sotile and Sotile rely on a 1999 survey conducted for the American Academy of Physician Executives (Table 1-2).[18]

Again, none of this material, I suspect, would surprise those in health care today. However, that this list is only part of the story and that the danger of burnout still exists as a serious threat to the psychological welfare of health care professionals and, in turn, those they serve make greater awareness of the form, causes, and description of compassion fatigue or burnout quite necessary. Too often we hear the following statements by nurses, physicians, and allied health professionals and take them as part of the territory of working in medical settings and not as symptoms that require vigilance:

- *Cynicism*: "I just see this as a job. Health care is not what it used to be. Nothing is going to change. People also ask me such trivial questions and burden me with stupid things."
- *Workaholism*: "I need to constantly check my email and phone mail even when I am not working on the weekend." "My husband and I need to earn a down payment for a house so I have to work more shifts than I'd like."
- *Isolation*: "I really don't feel part of things on the unit. The other nurses (physicians, EMS personnel, x-ray technicians, respiratory therapists, etc.) are nice people but I feel so different and isolated from them. I never discuss my work or personal life with any of them."
- *Boredom*: "I am so tired of doing the same thing every day. When I'm not killing myself, I'm bored to tears. If I hadn't so much invested in this field already, I would get out. I can't wait until the end of a shift."
- *Depletion:* "I feel it is taking me longer and longer to do less and less. I no longer feel the passion about the job as I did in the past. I am tired before I begin. I don't quite dread going into work but it certainly is getting to that point. All I think about is the job."
- *Conflict:* "Everything seems to get on my nerves now. I fight with the patients, am irritable with the staff, and am no fun

to be with at home. I also resent having to deal with patients'
families and feel that people are asking too much from me."

- *Arrogance:* "I wish I didn't have to deal with such incompetent
co-workers. Also, I wish the patients would just follow what
I tell them to do. One even had the nerve to ask for a second
opinion when I told her my diagnosis and treatment plan."
- *Helplessness:* "I am not sure I really can do anything to change
my situation. This is the workload I have to deal with, plain
and simple. Also, my sleeping is often disturbed, I have no time
for family and friends, my sinuses are always bothering me, and
I know I drink too much coffee in the morning and wine in
the evening."

Rather than only avoiding the dangers of burnout (as good as this may
be), professionals in health care should also take clear steps to prevent
acceleration of stress that is endemic to practice in the fields of medicine and nursing. To do this, several steps can be taken:

1. Appreciate the levels of burnout.
2. Take time to identify potential problem areas and review how
they are being addressed by developing a self-tailored *Personality Dysfunction Profile.*
3. Be aware of constructive approaches supervisors can take to
prevent or lessen secondary stress in the environment.

Levels of Burnout

The symptoms of chronic secondary stress include frustration, depression, apathy, helplessness, impatience, disengagement, emotional depletion, cynicism, hopelessness, a significant decline in one's professional
self-esteem and confidence, feeling overwhelmed, and anhedonia.[19]
However, for our purposes here, it may be helpful to break down the
possible progression of burnout, although doing this is somewhat artificial because there is much overlap between levels.

Among the ways burnout has been broken down, the levels provided by psychiatrist James Gill appear to be most helpful for those
in the medical, nursing, and allied health professions: "The *first level* is
characterized by signs and symptoms that are relatively mild, short in
duration and occur only occasionally [see Table 1-3]. . . . The *second level*

Table 1-3 Level 1—Daily Burnout: A Sampling of Key Signs and Symptoms

- Mentally fatigued at the end of the day
- Feeling unappreciated, frustrated, bored, tense, or angry as a result of a contact(s) with patients, colleagues, supervisors, superiors, assistants, or other potentially significant people
- Experiencing physical symptoms (e.g., headache, backache, upset stomach, etc.)
- Pace of day's activities and/or requirements of present tasks seem greater than personal or professional resources available
- Tasks required on job are repetitious, beyond the ability of the [caregiver], or require intensity on a continuous basis

Source: R. Wicks, R. Parsons, and D. Capps, *Clinical Handbook of Pastoral Counseling, Vol. 3* (Mahwah, NJ: Paulist Press, 2003), used with permission.

is reached when signs and symptoms have become *more stable, last longer* and are *tougher* to get rid of. . . . The *third level* is experienced when signs and symptoms have become *chronic* and a *physical illness* has developed"[20] [italics supplied].

As I have explained elsewhere, this "commonsense breakdown is very much in line with the medical model and there is some overlap between levels. While they could be applied to any physical or psychological constellation of symptoms and signs, they provide a reasonable way of delineating a breakdown of the burnout syndrome. The third level is self-explanatory. And in line with what is known about serious prolonged countertransference [feelings on the helpers' part toward patients and colleagues that have sources in their own past] . . . the signs, symptoms, and treatment are obvious. . . . If the [caregiver] is experiencing a life crisis and undergoing notable ongoing psychosomatic problems, then it means that preventive measures and self-administered treatments have failed. Psychological and medical assistance is necessary. This may mean entering or re-entering psychotherapy and obtaining, as advised by the therapist, medical help if necessary. Once this third level has been reached, the burnout is severe and remediation of the problem will likely take a good deal of time and effort."[21]

This is why it is essential to take preventative measures before reaching the point that we refer to here as "level 3." Because the seeds of burnout and the seeds of enthusiasm are in reality the same seeds, anyone who truly cares can expect to ride the waves of burnout—and occasionally get knocked down by a wave they missed! Basic steps to

Table 1-4 Level 1—Daily Burnout: Steps for Dealing with "Daily Burnout"

1. Correcting one's cognitive errors so there is a greater recognition when we are exaggerating or personalizing situations in an inappropriate, negative way
2. Having a variety of activities in one's daily schedule
3. Getting sufficient rest
4. Faithfully incorporating meditation [or quiet reflective time] into our daily schedule
5. Interacting on a regular basis with supportive friends
6. Being assertive
7. Getting proper nourishment and exercise
8. Being aware of the general principles set forth in the professional and self-help literature on stress management

Source: R. Wicks, R. Parsons, and D. Capps, *Clinical Handbook of Pastoral Counseling, Vol. 3* (Mahwah, NJ: Paulist Press, 2003), used with permission.

take in averting burnout (Table 1-4) should, in most cases, prevent many of the difficulties. Level 2 is "where the burnout problem has become more severe and intractable to brief interventions, a more profound effort is necessary. [See Table 1-5.] Central to such actions is a willingness to reorient priorities and take risks with one's style of dealing with the world, which for some reason is not working optimally. To accomplish this, frequently one's colleagues . . . [and] mentor need to become involved. Their support and insight for dealing with the distress being felt is needed. The uncomfortable steps taken to unlock oneself from social problems and the temptation to deal with them in a single unproductive way (repetition compulsion) requires all of the guidance and support one can obtain. In many cases, this also requires a break from work for a vacation or retreat in order to distance oneself from the work for a time so that revitalization and reorientation can occur."[22]

All medical and nursing professionals experience level 1 burnout throughout the year. It is part of the ups and downs of being in an intense profession. Most health care professionals also experience level 2 burnout at times, and some, unfortunately, level 3. This is why awareness of the ever-present challenges of stress, being as self-aware as possible, using this self-knowledge (see Chapter 2), developing a self-care protocol (see Chapter 4), and knowing what both psychology and spirituality from the perspective of the world's religions have to offer all of us—whether we are religious or not—as a way of strengthening one's "inner life" (see Chapter 3) are all essential. Beyond this, if we face stress

Table 1-5 Level 2—Minor Stress Becomes Distress: Some Major Signs and Symptoms

---

- Idealism and enthusiasm about being a [professional caregiver] waning; disillusionment about [work] . . . surfacing on a regular basis
- Experiencing a general loss of interest in the . . . field for a period of a month or longer
- Pervasive feeling of boredom, stagnation, apathy, and frustration
- Being ruled by schedule; seeing more and more patients; being no longer attuned to them; viewing them impersonally and without thought
- Losing criteria with which to judge the effectiveness of work . . .
- Inability to get refreshed by the other elements in one's life
- A loss of interest in professional resources (i.e., books, conferences, innovations, etc.) . . .
- Intermittent lengthy (week or more) periods of irritation, depression, and stress which do not seem to lift even with some effort to correct the apparent causes

---

Source: R. Wicks, R. Parsons, and D. Capps, *Clinical Handbook of Pastoral Counseling, Vol. 3* (Mahwah, NJ: Paulist Press, 2003), used with permission.

correctly, not only do we lessen the chances of it turning into extreme distress, we also are in a position to learn from it in a way that deepens us. However, this requires both the right type of knowledge and the humility to turn to others for help when we do not progress as we should—not an easy task when people in the health care setting often transfer onto us the sense that we are omnipotent, always strong, and usually right.

The reality, however, is far from the projections that are put onto us. We all have personalities-in-process and growing edges and are vulnerable to certain stresses, situations, and patient/colleague personality types. As a result, it would help immeasurably for us to be aware, through self-questioning, of the location of these vulnerable points so we are not caught unaware.

Personality Dysfunction Profile

Knowing what types of people and problems give you difficulty is the first step toward avoiding psychological vulnerability. Given this, the following questions may provide an avenue to helpful information with respect to individual stress points that are experienced by health care professionals:

- How do you deal with demanding patients?
- When young patients have a poor prognosis, what impact does this have on you?
- How do you blunt ("medicate") the pain you experience in medical/nursing practice?
- In what instances do you "dump" on co-workers or subordinates?
- What type of person "gets to you"?
- How do you handle unrealistic expectations of the medical/nursing staff and patients?
- What failures in the past haunt you now, and how have you learned from them?
- What procedures do you use to contain angry patients who direct their anger at the staff and stir up other patients in the waiting area?
- What prevents you from fully responding to life as a person and as a physician, nurse, or allied health professional?
- How do you handle unscheduled events in the day, such as multiple emergency add-ons (or, in the case of specialties like radiation oncology, machine breakdowns)?
- What are the things that you lie to yourself about or hide from co-workers, patients, and family?
- What most easily triggers your anger?
- About what are you most insecure?
- What is having the greatest negative impact on both your professional and personal life?
- How have you addressed the imbalances in your home life (with spouse, children, friends, etc.) given the intensity of nursing/medical practice?
- What are the ways you address problems in your department, such as understaffing/poor staffing, incompetence/poor work ethic, chronic complaining, rigidity, narrow compartmentalizing of responsibilities and not stepping beyond these roles, and overcompensating by some to deal with the weaknesses of others?

- Do you find yourself not listening to family or friends because you feel emotionally exhausted or because you feel that their problems are not as important as those of your patients?
- What themes run through your daydreams and night dreams?
- What recent cases produce in you the most guilt, resentment, or embarrassment?
- When are you the most bored with work, and what do you do about it?
- What are the coping mechanisms you use when you feel overwhelmed?

By addressing questions like these honestly and fully, you can begin to see the areas where you have progressed and developed effective coping skills. Other areas will need attention—sometimes *constant* attention—given our ingrained personality style. To ignore these areas is to court unnecessary stress. Even when you do not feel the stress, this can translate into a problem. As one professional told me when I questioned him about his problems with stress, "I don't think I really am usually under stress but I think I'm a carrier!" When we do induce stress in others, they in turn make life difficult for other workers, for family members, and so on, and this creates burnout contagion, which will eventually come back to haunt the "carrier" and decrease efficiency in the organization. That is why it is good to have some familiarity with the approaches necessary to lessen the stress in those around us.

Constructive Approaches for Clinical Supervisors to Use to Prevent or Lessen Chronic Secondary Stress

There are simple approaches that can be used both in the institution and in one's personal life to decrease the severity of chronic secondary stress (burnout). The following are sample steps to consider, especially if you are a clinical supervisor[23]:

- Provide opportunity for ventilation of complaints.
- Plan to remove "problem patients," who stir up other patients, from the earshot of other patients.
- Have constructive methods to curb inappropriate staff behavior by summarizing their action and letting the summary rather than you confront the person.

- Provide communication to staff of attempts made by physicians to improve work environment so they realize their critiques are being addressed whenever possible.
- Spontaneously buy lunches when spirits are high or low.
- Compliment staff in front of colleagues, patients, and supervisors.
- Try to "keep it light" whenever possible.
- Encourage creative problem-solving within staff's sphere of responsibility to encourage initiative and avoid morale-destroying impact of micro-organization.
- To avoid a sense of not being heard, appreciated, or regarded well or of feeling discounted—one of the greatest stresses on nurses—encourage the unit director and physicians "to be aware of and accept nurses' practical sensibilities and innovative ideas as well as their caring and compassionate nature, all of which will greatly benefit physicians and patients alike."[24]

The above are obviously only a sampling of simple approaches that one can use. They are offered to stimulate your creativity in this area. The important thing is to begin to become more aware of the approaches you are already using that work well. In addition, it would help to broaden that repertoire by using these suggestions and to take a page from the approach notebook of other successful physician/nurse/allied health managers to lessen the possibility of chronic secondary stress. Health care settings can be psychologically toxic. There are many environmental factors there and within our personal milieu that can increase stress. Physician Sidha Sambandan, from the United Kingdom, recognizes this in a chapter on burnout:

> We experience external stressors in our daily life, including major life events and the daily hassles of life. Other factors are workload and other loads. They are only triggers, and not the only cause of the stress syndrome. Major factors that act as stressors in the professional context are as follows:
> - *Information overload.* The rapid advance in information technology has resulted in an information explosion, accessible by anybody—both patients and doctors. The globe has shrunk with the advent of electronic mail and the worldwide web. This has necessitated new skills for the medical profession—the ability to search, select, and critically

appraise the information. This has to be applied to practice, which is the ultimate purpose of the exercise.

- *Rapid advances in medical technology.* These have necessitated the development of new knowledge and skills in diagnostic and therapeutic procedures, as well as making the concept of rationing much more explicit, with a risk that it could erode the doctor-patient relationship.

- *Expanding workload, within shrinking financial and material resources.* Increasing consumerism has resulted in both increasing demands and expectations from patients. In addition, doctors find themselves also accountable to both managers and consumers, with the attendant stresses that inevitably follow.

- *Increasing patient expectations and demands.* Patient expectations and demands have increased over the past few years. The public is better "informed" and, in the [United Kingdom], media publicity about [some examples of] substandard practice . . . has results in the demand for greater professional regulation by the stake-holders and the public.[25]

Another treatment of the topic, this time from the United States, points out that "Stress in nursing often leads to burn-out, the three major causes of which are (1) a mismatch between efforts and results . . . leading to disappointment and frustration, (2) a mismatch between nurse and environment . . . leading to role ambiguity and conflict, and (3) a mismatch between people . . . leading to interpersonal conflict. The issue in all three is control or, more specifically, the discrepancy between the nurse's need to control events, environment, and people and his or her inability to do so. . . . The reality for many nurses is that they feel powerless to change their circumstances. . . . Finally, contextual stressors and interpersonal conflicts, not to mention actual discrimination in work situations, are the proverbial straws that break the camel's back."[26]

This is only a sample of the types of environmental factors that face nurses, physicians, and other health professionals, so anything that can be done to deal with these sources of stress must be done. We realize this even more clearly when we recognize that in addition to chronic stress, there is an acute counterpart with which we must be familiar.

Acute Secondary Stress: Vicarious Posttraumatic
Stress Disorder

Psychologist Jeffrey Kottler said about the threats to his personal sense
of well-being that were a byproduct of his work: "Never mind that we
catch [our patients'] colds and flus, what about their pessimism, negativity. . . . Words creep back to haunt us. Those silent screams remain deaf-
ening."[27] What he is speaking about here is the destabilization of one's
own personality as a result of constant treatment of the severe psychological and physical trauma experienced by others.

Vicarious posttraumatic stress is a great danger today in health care
settings. Not only must physicians, nurses, and other health professionals
deal with medical emergencies, they also must increasingly ease the suffering that patients experience due to the psychic trauma arising from
abuse, rape and other physical assaults, and terrorism. When this mixes
with the stress that health care professionals experience in their lives—
including marital, financial, personal, and world instability—the result
is quite psychologically toxic. Unrecognized, it could lead to severe
impairment or a psychological "grayness" in how one experiences life,
as well as a resultant inadequate treatment of patients due to one's emotional state.

One of the most sensible approaches to recognizing, limiting, avoiding, and even learning from the onset of vicarious PTSD is to conduct
daily debriefings with yourself. A second approach is to have an organized way to question yourself to uncover the presence and/or duration
of clusters of PTSD signs and symptoms. These two approaches go hand
in hand. As I noted previously:

> Persons in the helping professions . . . at times lose distance
> and are temporarily swept away by the expectations, needs,
> painful experiences, and negativity of others. More than most
> people, they are confronted with negativity and sadness. Yet,
> they are educated to pick up these signs as early as possible so
> they are not unnecessarily dragged down. We can learn much
> from how they avoid losing perspective or regain it when they
> temporarily lose their way. The distance they value can help us
> deal with the pain of others.
>
> There is much to remembering the Russian proverb:
> "When you live next to the cemetery, you can't cry for every-

one who dies." Most of us, whether we are professional helpers or not, tend to personalize too much. We absorb the sadness, anxiety, and negativity of those around us. Sometimes we even feel this is expected of us. . . . As we listen to stories of terrible things that happen [or observe them] . . . we catch some of their futility, fear, vulnerability, and hopelessness rather than experiencing mere frustration or concern. We learn that no matter how professionally prepared we are, we are not immune to the psychological and spiritual dangers that arise in living a full life of involvement with others. I remember learning this the hard way myself.

In 1994 I did a psychological debriefing of some of the relief workers evacuated from Rwanda's bloody civil war. I interviewed each person and gave them an opportunity to tell their stories. As they related the horrors they had experienced, they seemed to be grateful for an opportunity to ventilate. They recounted the details again and again, relating their feelings as well as descriptions of the events which triggered them. Their sense of futility, their feelings of guilt, their sense of alienation, their experiences with emotional outbursts, all came to the fore.

In addition to listening, I gave them handouts on what to possibly expect down the road (problems sleeping, difficulties trusting and relating to others, flashbacks and the like). As I moved through the process of debriefing and providing information so they could have a frame of reference for understanding their experiences, I thought to myself, "This is going pretty well." Then, something happened that shifted my whole experience.

In the course of one of the final interviews, one of the relief workers related stories of how certain members of the Hutu tribe raped and dismembered their Tutsi foes. Soon, I noticed I was holding onto my chair for dear life. I was doing what some young people call "white knuckling it."

After the session, I did what I usually do after an intense encounter . . . a countertransferential review. (If time doesn't permit then, I do it at the end of the day—every day.) In doing this, I get in touch with my feelings by asking myself: What made me sad? Overwhelmed me? Sexually aroused me?

Made me extremely happy or even confused me? Being bru-
tally honest with myself, I try to put my finger on the pulse
of my emotions.

The first thing that struck me about this particular session
was the tight grip I had on the chair as the session with the
relief worker progressed. "What was I feeling when I did this?
Why did I do this?"

It didn't take me long to realize that their terrible stories
had broken through my defenses and normal sense of distance
and detachment. I was holding onto the chair because quite
simply, I was frightened to death that if I didn't I would be
pulled into the vortex of darkness myself.

That recognition alone helped lessen the pain and my fearful uneasiness. I then proceeded with a . . . countertransferential review . . . used by therapists . . . to prevent the slide into
unnecessary darkness and to learn—and thus benefit—from
the events for the day.[28]

The questions we can ask ourselves to determine whether vicarious
PTSD may well be present are fairly straightforward (Table 1-6). (The
guidelines of the profile for this syndrome noted in the American Psychiatric Association's *Diagnostic and Statistical Manual of Mental Disorders* provide additional assistance as to what may constitute a significant
problem in this area.)

The essential frame of reference to use in understanding this self-
questioning is that having these symptoms is no more a sign of personal
weakness than is having the symptoms of any medical disorder. This is
important to note at the outset so that self-blame, self-debasement, or
bravado does not prevent a careful self-examination—especially after
a particularly difficult patient/clinical encounter. Working with young
victims of abuse, pediatric oncology patients, victims of brutal rape, or
severe burn patients over a period of time would take a toll on anyone.

To ensure that the medical or nursing professional takes this
approach, I point them to the following general principles to keep in
mind when seeking self-understanding after a single or series of traumatic encounters:

1. Be as nonjudgmental and accepting of yourself as you would
   in dealing with those you treat who have undergone a traumatic event.

Table 1-6 Questions to Ask to Uncover Vicarious PTSD

If one or more of the following symptoms or signs have lasted longer than 1 month and are presently interfering in your personal and professional life, care must be taken to consider that the result of being constantly exposed to persons who have experienced trauma may be having a vicarious impact on the health care provider:

1. Do you find that you are re-experiencing past traumatic events?
   a. Nightmares
   b. Intrusive thoughts
   c. Flashbacks to events
   d. Reliving events
   e. Association of events in present with past trauma or the traumatic experiences of others

2. Are you experiencing a blunting of affect, numbing, loss of feelings, or tendency to avoid reminders of a past traumatic event?
   a. Feeling a sense of detachment or restriction of range of emotions
   b. Avoiding thoughts, feelings, conversations, people, or activities that are reminders of past trauma
   c. Having memory lacunae with respect to past trauma-laden events
   d. Having morbid view of the future (e.g., expected shortened length or outlook of remainder of health care career, life span, family life, etc.)

3. Do you have a heightened or exaggerated sense of arousal?
   a. Hyperalert or usually feeling "on guard"
   b. Pronounced startle reaction
   c. Irritability or a "short emotional fuse"
   d. Problems concentrating, sleeping, eating, or enjoying normal activities that previously brought you pleasure or provided a sense of mastery

4. Do you experience dramatic alterations in your outlook or world view?
   a. Personal sense of safety/trust is fragile
   b. Positive view of the human condition is absent
   c. View of one's own power, independence, and self-confidence/esteem is now questioned
   d. Awareness of cruelty or fragility of life (given the experiences of colleagues or patients whom you have treated) is often present in a depressing, somewhat frightening way
   e. Feelings of shame, guilt, depression, or worthlessness are increasingly present

5. Have you begun to demonstrate symptoms or exaggerated signs of antisocial/asocial behavior that were not present before the overwhelming/ongoing exposure to your patients' trauma?
   a. Dangerous behavior (e.g., sexual promiscuity, erratic/aggressive/careless driving patterns, fiscal irresponsibility, poor treatment plan development, etc.)
   b. Extreme irresponsibility in one's personal and professional lives
   c. Alcohol abuse, illegal drug use, self-medication, criminal behavior

Table 1-6 *(continued)*

6. Are your basic interpersonal relations becoming dramatically affected?
    a. Suspicious, cynical, or hypercritical style now present
    b. Boundary violations with patients and staff
    c. Loss of interest in activities at home and/or work
    d. Poor patterns of self-care resulting in alterations in interactions with others
    e. Lack of availability

2. Constantly keep in mind that the symptoms you are experiencing as a result of the traumatic encounter are related to the experiences themselves rather than to an inherent personality weakness or lack of personality strength in oneself.
3. Know that when you are dealing with trauma on an ongoing basis as part of the work you do, then dealing with the symptoms and dangers of vicarious PTSD on an ongoing basis— rather than a once-and-for-all event—is to be expected.
4. Sharing your feelings and concerns with others is clinically wise; those who seek to go it alone either wind up leaving the field or acting out in unhealthy ways (alcoholism, overdetachment, promiscuity, etc.).
5. Grieving losses along with the family of patients (especially young persons) is a task that is periodically necessary for professionals in health care.

In some cases, a more formal type of critical incident stress debriefing (CISD) may be needed. Jeffrey T. Mitchell and the Holeman Group have done extensive work in this area. In a basic adaptation of the process for emergency medical services personnel, Seaward notes the following summary:

> Dynamics During an Incident
> The first aspect of CISD involves both on-scene support services and defusing stress immediately after the event. A debriefing team provides on-scene support services to assist obviously distressed personnel. Defusings are described as "short unstructured debriefings" to reduce acute stress by discussing the details of the event. This session is typically conducted

upon return to the station and is short (about 30–60 minutes). Demobilizations, like defusings, take place immediately after an incident, particularly a large-scale incident; however, in contrast to the defusing or debriefing, personnel are not obligated to discuss the incident. Talking is optional in this half-hour session, after which all personnel are encouraged to rest either at the station or at home before resuming their routine duties.

CISD Dynamics After an Incident

Because emotional reactions can be so intense in the first 24 hours after a critical incident, a formal CISD is typically scheduled by a CISD team several days after the critical incident. A formal CISD is both a psychological and educational support group discussion under the guidance of a well-prepared CISD team. The purpose of CISD is to enable personnel to return to their routine lives as quickly as possible. This procedure has seven phases.

First, a formal CISD is initiated with an introduction by the CISD team members. Personnel are reminded that all material is confidential. Second, facts of the incident are discussed as staff members describe in their own words what happened at the scene. Third, the debriefing team leader initiates a discussion called a *thought phase* to help staff members to personalize their experience. Rather than facts, they describe how they personally experienced the event. The fourth phase is called the *reaction phase*, in which personnel share what they consider to be the worst part of the event. It is this phase that is most cathartic in dealing with emotions triggered by the incident. The *symptom phase* is the fifth step in the process in which the team leader asks personnel to identify stress symptoms at three distinct times: initially during the incident, three to five days after the incident, and later. The symptom phase is followed by the *teaching phase*, in which group members are taught several stress management techniques . . . grief processing and communication skills that can be used with spouses and significant support group members. The last phase is the *reentry phase*, in which group members are given a chance to ask questions. After any discussion, the CISD is concluded. At this time, if the

CISD team members feel that one or more of the participants might benefit from counseling, referrals are made.[29]

Another important factor in having a healthy attitude in dealing with *vicarious* PTSD in yourself is appreciating a bit more about PTSD in the general population, and it is to this topic that we turn next.

What Is Posttraumatic Stress Disorder?

Although we hear a lot about PTSD today—especially after the September 11th attacks on the World Trade Center and the Pentagon—it is far from a new phenomenon. An overview is provided by Foy, Drescher, Fitz, and Kennedy:

> Surviving a life-threatening personal experience often produces intense psychological reactions in the forms of intrusive thoughts about the experience and fear-related avoidance of reminders. In the first few weeks following a traumatic experience these patterns are found in most individuals and thus seem to represent a natural response mechanism for psychological adaptation to a life-changing event. Persistence of this reaction pattern at troublesome levels beyond a three-month period, however, indicates that the natural psychological adjustment process, like mourning in the bereaved, has been derailed. At that point the psychological reactions natural in the first few weeks become symptoms of PTSD. In other words, PTSD may be seen as the persistence of a natural process beyond its natural time frame for resolutions.
>
> The cardinal features of PTSD are trauma-specific symptoms of intrusion, avoidance, and physical arousal. The primary requirement is the presence of. . . . A life-threatening event, such as serious injury in a traffic accident, would satisfy this criterion, while the expected death of a loved one from natural causes would not. The current diagnostic system then groups PTSD symptoms into three additional categories. [It] includes the presence in some form of persistent intrusive thoughts and feelings. Recurrent distressing dreams or flashbacks while awake about the traumatic experience are

examples. . . . [The second category] represents the presence
of avoidance symptoms associated with the trauma, such as
avoiding driving following a severe traffic accident or fear of
sexual relations following sexual assault. More subtle forms of
avoidance would be general numbing of responsiveness or the
absence of strong feelings about the trauma. . . . [The final]
reflects the presence of symptoms of increased physical arousal
and hyper-vigilance. Feelings of panic may be experienced in
situations similar to the trauma; for example, combat veterans
with PTSD may show powerful startle reactions to loud noises
that resemble gunshots or explosions.

The medical history of PTSD can be traced back to studies of human reactions to trauma in the nineteenth century
by German psychiatrists who discovered the similarities in the
clinical courses of survivors of mining accidents and accidents
which involved toxic exposure.[30] Two major developments at
that time stimulated investigations into what was then called
post-traumatic neurosis. The initial spark of medical interest
in the subject was ignited by a series of wars, including the
Civil War in America and the two World Wars in Europe. Early
conceptions of combat-related PTSD by physicians working
with veterans of World War I presented it as "shell shock," a
consequence of organic dysfunction rather than a psychological process. This formulation arose from use in World War I of
both chemical agents and explosives of a power that previously
had been unimaginable.

The second impetus was the emergence of social programs
in several countries which began to provide compensation for
work-related or military service-related disabilities. The early
description of traumatic reactions as "compensation reactions"
referred to a perceived rise in numbers of victims seeking res-
titution after the first compensation laws were introduced in
Europe. . . . This phenomenon presented an example of the
tendency to relate symptoms of a trauma reaction to some
process other than exposure to intense trauma itself.

While early views of post-traumatic reactions reflected
the assumption that various types of trauma produced similar reactions, studies in the past twenty years have tended to
be trauma-specific in their focus. Thus, labels for PTSD such

as battle fatigue, rape trauma syndrome, and disaster survivor syndrome have developed in the literature.[31] However, most recently, studies have shown similarities among several survivor groups, including combat,[32] rape, domestic violence,[33] childhood sexual abuse,[34] childhood physical abuse,[35] transportation accidents,[36] and natural disasters.[37] [Since 9/11, terrorism has been added to the list.]

Common elements of traumatic experience include being physically and psychologically overwhelmed by a life-threatening event which is beyond the victim's prediction and control. To understand such complex reaction patterns requires the integration of findings from both biology and psychology. Thus, current perspectives on the nature of PTSD include contributions from several approaches, including biological, behavioral, cognitive,[38] and integrative.[39]

From a biological perspective a number of studies in the past ten years have been conducted with Vietnam combat veterans with PTSD to examine their physiological reactions to combat trauma reminders or cues. Results from these studies have been consistent in showing large heart rate increases in most combat veterans with PTSD when they were exposed to combat cues. Other biological studies have also shown that combat veterans with PTSD have experienced changes in their central nervous systems so that they are overly sensitive to startle-producing noises. Studies are currently being conducted to determine whether these biological features are also applicable to PTSD associated with other types of trauma. Since these physical features of PTSD are almost universally described as painfully distressing in nature, this biological reactivity may be a critical element in the onset of social irritability and withdrawal in PTSD victims.

Contributions from behavioral psychology help in understanding how PTSD symptoms develop. Pavlovian conditioning occurs at the time of the trauma so that the overpowering feelings of life-threat and helplessness are paired with other cues present (which are not life-threatening). By this learning process these cues acquire the potential for evoking extreme fear when they are encountered later. The survivor also learns that escaping from these cues terminates the distressing fear.

Planning life activities to avoid painful reminders, an example of instrumental learning, may become a preferred coping strategy since it reduces the painful exposure to trauma reminders.

From a cognitive psychology perspective, the meaning which the survivor attaches to the traumatic experience may play an important role in PTSD. Perceptions of helplessness associated with the traumatic experience may serve to immobilize survivors' more active coping efforts, thereby serving to maintain PTSD symptoms.

While these approaches are helpful in explaining possible mechanisms for the development of PTSD, they do not explain why some individuals exposed to intense trauma do not develop enduring PTSD symptoms. In order to address this issue an integrative approach is necessary which includes additional factors beyond biological reactivity, Pavlovian and instrumental learning, and symbolic meaning. In our integrative model of PTSD the experience of an overwhelming biological reaction during a life-threatening traumatic event lays the necessary foundation for the development of PTSD through behavioral and cognitive mechanisms of learning. However, other factors serve to mediate between exposure to trauma and the development of PTSD symptoms. Thus, an integrative approach to understanding PTSD includes the interaction between traumatic experiences and other non-trauma factors to account for the development or non-development of PTSD.[40]

Once again, knowing as much as you can about PTSD is essential not only for patient care and referral but also for your own health and the welfare of your colleagues and those whom you supervise. When vicarious PTSD disrupts the medical professional's frame of reference, the results will change his or her world view, sense of professional and personal identity, and spiritual, psychological, and philosophical outlooks. The negative ripple effect may lead to personal alienation from friends and long-term coworkers and even in the relationship one has with oneself. It can cause an abrupt and inappropriate job change and a dramatic alteration of one's personality style with and approach to others (i.e., inability to modulate emotions). Extremes such as absenteeism or overinvolvement may not only cause personal problems but also be bad role models for other members of the treatment team. Consequently, as in the case of chronic secondary stress, awareness of this potential problem is essential. And, building on this awareness of the challenges of stress, knowing how to develop a self-care protocol, being able to increase one's ongoing level of self-understanding (even in, especially in, difficult situations that may involve failure and loss of life), and knowing ways to strengthen your inner life are also essential. Accordingly, it is to these topics that we turn next and devote the majority of this book.

Objectives of Chapter One

- Know definition and contributing causes of chronic second-ary stress (also known as "compassion fatigue" or "burnout")
- Appreciate the different signs, symptoms, and levels of burn-out
- Be aware of constructive steps you can take as supervisors to lessen secondary stress in the environment
- Be familiar with the types of questions to ask yourself to deter-mine your own "Personality Dysfunction Profile"
- Have a basic understanding of posttraumatic stress syndrome (PTSD)
- Possess fluency with an approach to take in questioning/infor-mally debriefing yourself and others when PTSD or vicarious PTSD symptoms and signs first become evident

Additional Books to Consider

The Sotiles' book *The Resilient Physician* is the most recent and com-prehensive book on physician stress. It is a treasure trove of information on the topic. The chapter you have just read provides a good preface to the extended treatment of a number of the topics covered in *The Resil-ient Physician*. Chapter 3 on "The Psychology of Physicians," Chapter 4 on "Stress Resilience," and Chapters 6 and 7 on "Conflict Self-Assess-ment" and "Anger Management" are especially helpful and informative. This book is truly a rich resource for those wishing to read further on physicians and stress. I also found *Not Another Guide to Stress in General*

Practice, edited by David Haslam, to be very practical. It is one of several books from the United Kingdom published by Radcliffe Medical Press in Oxford, and it is filled with useful suggestions by practitioners in the field. Other titles include *Survival Skills* by Ruth Chambers, *The GP's Guide to Personal Development Plans* by Amar Rughani, and *The PCG Team Builder: Creating and Maintaining Effective Team Working* by Roy Lilley with Gareth Davies and Bill Cain. (Other Radcliffe titles are listed in "Bibliography" at the end of this book.)

In the nursing area, most of the books on stress were published in the 1980s. Of them, the ones I believe still have great relevance today include: Smythe's *Surviving Nursing*, Roy Bailey and Margaret Clarke's *Stress and Coping in Nursing*, and James Humphrey's *Stress in the Nursing Profession*. Other titles are listed in "Bibliography." Possibly a better or an adjunctive approach is to review the more current treatment of the topic of stress and   nursing in the clinical and research papers that have been published in the past 10 years. Key selections from this literature are contained in the bibliography at the end of this book.

A general title worth reviewing as well is Figley's *Compassion Fatigue*. It is a fine overview of the topic of chronic secondary stress. You may wish to supplement it as well with Foa's book on PTSD or any other recent work on the topic, as they are, for the most part, uniformly sound because this is a very focused area.

Notes

1. R. Bode, *First You Have to Row a Little Boat* (New York: Warner, 1993), 49.

2. T. Shanafelt, K. Bradley, J. Wipf, and A. Back, "Burnout and Self-Reported Patient Care in an Internal Medicine Residency Program," *Annals of Internal Medicine* 136, 5, (2002): 358–367.

3. L. Clever, "Who Is Sicker: Patients—or Residents? Residents' Distress and the Care of Patients, *Annals of Internal Medicine*, 136, 5 (2002), 391.

4. L. Sanders, *The Case of Lucy Bending* (New York: Putnam, 1982), 42.

5. McLuhan M, source unknown.

6. E. Smythe, *Surviving Nursing* (Los Angeles: Western Schools, 1994), 27.

7. Personal communication with B. Eanes, August 11, 2004.

8. J. Edelwich and A. Brodsky, *Burnout* (New York: Human Sciences Press, 1980), 14.

9. H. Freudenberger, "Impaired Clinicians: Coping with Burnout," in P. A. Keller and L. Ritt (Eds.), *Innovations in Clinical Practice: A Sourcebook, Vol. 3* (Sarasota, FL: Professional Resource Exchange, 1984), 223.

10. J. H. Pfifferling, "Cultural Antecedents Promoting Professional Impairment," in C. D. Scott and J. Hawk (Eds.), *Heal Thyself: The Health of Health Care Professionals* (New York: Brunner Mazel Publishers, 1986), 3–18.

11. J. Gill, "Burnout: A Growing Threat in Ministry," *Human Development*, 1 (2) Summer (1980), 21, 24, 25.

12. R. Wicks, "Countertransference and Burnout in Pastoral Counseling," in R. Wicks, R. Parsons, and D. Capps (Eds.), *Clinical Handbook of Pastoral Counseling, Vol. 3* (Mahwah, NJ: Paulist Press, 2003), 336.

13. L. Gunderson, "Physician Burnout," *Annals of Internal Medicine* 135 (2001), 145–148.

14. W. M. Sotile and M. O. Sotile, *The Medical Marriage: Sustaining Healthy Relationships for Physicians and Their Families* (Chicago, IL: American Medical Association, 2000).

15. W. M. Sotile and M. O. Sotile, *The Resilient Physician* (Chicago, IL: American Medical Association, 2002), 10.

16. P. Sullivan and L. Burke, "Results from CMA's Huge 1998 Physician Survey Point to a Dispirited Profession," *Canadian Medical Association Journal* 159 (1998): 525–529.

17. W. H. Auden, "Introduction," in Dag Hammarskjold, *Markings* (New York: Knopf, 1976), ix.

18. C. A. Aschenbrener and C. T. Siders, "Managing Low-to-Mid Intensity Conflict in the Health Care Setting," *The Physician Executive* 25 (1999): 44–50.

19. See Robert J. Wicks (2003), Skovholt (2001), Maslach and Jackson (1981), James Gill (1980), and Baker (2003) in Bibliography.

20. J. Gill, *Op. Cit.* (1980), 22–23.

21. R. Wicks, *Op. Cit.* (2003), 337.

22. R. Wicks, *Ibid.* 338.

23. I am grateful to Sally Cheston, M.D., for her suggestions in this section.

24. This last point was suggested by Beverly Eanes, Ph.D., R.N.

25. S. Sambandan, "Burnout," in D. Haslam (Ed.), *Not Another Guide to Stress in Practice*, 2nd ed. (Oxford, UK: Radcliffe Medical Press, 2002), 23–24.

26. E. Smythe, *Op. Cit.* (1994), 31.

27. J. Kottler, *On Being a Therapist* (San Francisco, CA: Jossey-Bass, 1986), 8.

28. R. Wicks, *Riding the Dragon* (Notre Dame, IN: Sorin Books, 2002), 54–56, 109.

29. B. Seward, *Managing Stress in Emergency Medical Services* (Sudbury, MA: American Academy of Orthopaedic Surgeons/Jones and Bartlett, 2000), 9.

30. L. C. Kolb, "A Critical Survey of Hypotheses Regarding Posttraumatic Stress Disorders in Light of Recent Research Findings," *Journal of Traumatic Stress* I (1988): 291–304.

31. E. B. Foa, G. Steketee, and B. Olasov Rothbam, "Behavioral/Cognitive Conceptualizations of Post-traumatic Stress Disorder," *Behavior Therapy* 20 (1989): 155–176.

32. D. W. Foy, R. C. Sipprelle, D. B. Rueger, and E. M. Carroll, "Etiology of Posttraumatic Stress Disorder in Vietnam Veterans: Analysis of Premilitary, Military, and Combat Exposure Influences," *Journal of Consulting and Clinical Psychology* 52 (1984): 79–87; T. M. Keane, J. A. Fairbank, J. M. Caddell, and R. T. Zimering, "Therapy Reduces Symptoms of PTSD in Vietnam Combat Veterans," *Behavior Therapy* 20 (1989): 245–260.

33. B. Houskamp, and D. W. Foy, "The Assessment of PTSD in Battered Women," *Journal of Interpersonal Violence* (in press).

34. J. Briere, *Therapy for Adults Molested as Children: Beyond Survival* (New York: Springer, 1989).

35. R. T. Ammerman, J. E. Cassisi, M. Hersen, and V. B. Van-Hasselt, "Consequences of Physical Abuse and Neglect in Children," *Clinical Psychology Review* 6 (1986): 291–310.

36. R. McCaffrey and J. Fairbank, "Behavioral Assessment and Treatment of Accident-Related Posttraumatic Stress Disorder: Two Case Studies," *Behavior Therapy* 16 (1985) 406–416.

37. B. L. Green, M. C. Grace, and G. C. Gleser, "Identifying Survivors at Risk: Long-term Impairment Following the Beverly Hills Supper Club Fire," *Journal of Consulting & Clinical Psychology* 53 (1985): 672–678.

38. E. Foa, G. Stekelee, and B. Olasov Rothbaum, "Behavioral/Cognitive Conceptualizations of Post-traumatic Stress Disorder," *Behavior Therapy* 20 (1989): 155–176.

39. D. W. Foy, S. Osato, B. Houskamp, and D. Neumann, "Etiology Factors in Posttraumatic Stress Disorder," in P. Saigh (Ed.), *Posttraumatic Stress Disorder: A Behavioral Approach to Assessment and Treatment* (Oxford, UK: Pergamon Press, in press).

40. D. Foy, K. Drescher, A. Fitz, and K. Kennedy, "Post-Traumatic Stress Disorders," in R. Wicks, R. Parsons, and D. Capps (Eds.), *Clinical Handbook of Pastoral Counseling, Vol. 3* (Mahwah, NJ: Paulist Press, 2003), 274–277.

TWO

"Riding the Dragon"

*Enhancing Self-Knowledge and Self-Talk
in the Health Care Professional*

In a foreword to a book on identifying and avoiding defensive patterns in working with patients, Dame Lesley Southgate wrote, "The missing pieces about the failure of some doctors to incorporate best practice into the consultation may be addressed by paying attention to what the doctor is feeling rather than what he/she knows."[1] If acute and chronic secondary stress is to be limited and one's personal and professional well-being is to be enhanced, self-knowledge and the enlightened behavior that it should give rise to are not a nicety in medical/nursing practice; they must be a given. Personal discipline and self-control are essential in nursing and medicine, as they are for all professionals responsible for the care for others. In the behavioral sciences, this is referred to as "self-regulation." In a book for psychologists on self-care, Baker writes, "*Self-regulation*, a term used in both behavioral and dynamic psychology, refers to the conscious and less conscious management of our physical and emotional impulses, drives and anxieties."[2] She then goes on to warn:

> Managing our affect, stimulation, and energy as we navigate
> our professional and personal lives, as well as our relationships
> with self and others, is no easy task. To regulate mood and
> affect, we must learn how to both proactively, constructively
> manage dysphoric affect (such as anxiety and depression)

47

and adaptively defuse or "metabolize" intense, charged emotional experiences to lessen the risk of becoming emotionally flooded and overwhelmed.

However, as Coster and Schwebel point out, if we are to "manage" ourselves or "regulate" our behavior, obviously sound self-awareness must be present.[3] Nowhere is this more necessary than in the medical setting.

Self-awareness is especially important for persons working in high-stress settings that require great intelligence and high standards. In such professions, "perfectionism and its associated demon, fear of failure," as Block recognizes, can be quite dangerous to the types of persons attracted to health care.[4] He goes on to point out the following:

> Health professionals are held, and for the most part hold themselves, to extremely high standards of performance. It is believed that they should always be at the peak of technical proficiency, emotionally available, straightforward, clear, and compassionate. The rewards for this are high status, admiration and respect. Lapses are in two directions: cynicism and money grubbing, or despair, feelings of failure, and disgrace. This latter triad is often associated with the more frank and overt symptomatic breakdown into addiction and substance abuse.[5]

It is very easy to lose one's way—even from the very beginning of one's journey in professional health care. Harvard University psychiatrist Robert Coles, in reflecting on his years in medical school, shares a story that aptly illustrates this:

> I was in medical school in Columbia and not enjoying it much. Kept complaining about it to my mother, and she said that what I needed was to go down and work at a [New York City] soup kitchen for Dorothy Day instead of complaining. I understood what my mother was getting at. She used to say that there are things more important than the troubles you're having, and there are people who might help you to understand that and especially help you to get some distance from your complaining and from the rather privileged position of being a medical student. The long and short of it is, I eventually went down there and met Dorothy Day.[6]

Unfortunately, this problem does not end with graduation. Loss of perspective remains a danger through one's career if time is not taken to reflect on one's personal and professional lives. The following anecdote on how easy it was for a seasoned neurologist to lose a sense of what was important illustrates this well. He demonstrates, as did Cole, that sometimes even when you are dealing with life and death on a daily basis, it takes someone from your circle of friends or family to remind you how quickly all of us can blow things out of proportion when we do not take time out to reflect on our feelings, thoughts, beliefs, and behavior.

> The following letter, written by a first-year college student to her father during the middle of her second semester, delightfully points [out how easy it is to lose perspective no matter how delicate and important one's work is]. Prior to receiving this note, her father was totally preoccupied with her "success" in college. He was worried because she didn't do well in her first semester and was concerned she would fail out during the second semester—and take his money with her! He had forgotten, as many of us parents do, that performance in courses is only a partial measure of learning; moreover, there is much more to the total college experience than just grades.

> Despite her youth, this woman knew this better than he, and so taught him an important lesson on perspective. On the front page of her note it said:

> Dear Dad,
>
> Everything is going well here at college this semester, so you can stop worrying. I am very, very happy now . . . you would love Ichabod. He is a wonderful, wonderful man and our first three months of marriage have been blissful.
>
> And more good news Dad. The drug rehab program we are both in just told us that the twins that are due soon will not be addicted at birth.
>
> Having read this, her father then turned the page with trepidation. On the other side of the note it said:
>
> Now, Dad, there actually is no Ichabod. I'm not married nor pregnant. And I haven't ever abused drugs. But I did get a "D" in chemistry, so keep things in perspective![7]

It is very easy to move through life—even the most service oriented of lives—in such a compulsive, driven way that we feel out of control. When we take out time to reflect on who we are and what we are doing, we often see how "unfree" we have become in so many ways. In his most classic work, physician and Russian spiritual leader Anthony Bloom puts it in a way that is easy to image:

> There is a passage in Dickens' *Pickwick Papers* which is a very good description of my life and probably also of your lives. Pickwick goes to the club. He hires a cab and on the way he asks innumerable questions. Among the questions, he says, "Tell me, how is it possible that such a mean and miserable horse can drive such a big and heavy cab?" The cabbie replies "It's not a question of the horse, Sir, it's a question of the wheels," and Mr. Pickwick says "What do you mean?" The cabbie answers "You see, we have a magnificent pair of wheels which are so well oiled that it is enough for the horse to stir a little for the wheels to begin to turn and then the poor horse must run for its life."[8]

Bloom then adds by way of commentary on this: "Take the way we live most of the time. We are not the horse that pulls, we are the horse that runs away from the cab in fear of its life." The bottom line is that you can count on losing perspective and deluding yourself if time is not devoted to reflection on your thoughts, behavior, and affects. But it is not easy to be honest with yourself.

Zen master Shunryu Suzuki once cautioned his students, "When you are fooled by something else, the damage will not be so big. But when you are fooled by yourself, it is fatal."[9] In health care, this is a particular danger. In a book on the dynamics of being a woman physician, the author wrote, "What's good about medicine is that there is always something to do, so you don't have to think about your problem." Then, she added: "What's bad about medicine is that you don't have to think about your problems *enough*"[10] [italics added].

A medical oncologist was sharing his thoughts about whether a certain drug was inducing retinopathy in one of his patients. He said that in his search of the literature he found, in one study, the finding for this was positive. However, as he studied it further he found that the subjects in this study were all older than 60 years, so he was unsure whether that variable or the drug was responsible for the vision impairment. This type of close examination of studies is something we applaud and possibly expect of medical professionals. They are encouraged to do this in medical, nursing, and other professional health care educational programs. However, very few of these programs also encourage these practitioners to use the same seriousness in going the extra mile in examining themselves.

This is not surprising because even in psychotherapy, real self-knowledge is sometimes elusive. Donald Brazier reflects this reality in a book advocating the use of an integration of Zen with psychotherapy when he notes,

> These days . . . we are apt to seek out a therapist to . . . help us get the dragon back into its cave. Therapists of many schools will oblige in this, and we will thus be returned to what Freud called 'ordinary unhappiness' and, temporarily, heave a sigh of relief, our repressions working smoothly once again. Zen, by contrast offers dragon-riding lessons, for the few who are sufficiently intrepid.[11]

Given the personal psychological dangers to medical practitioners and their patients when they are not self-aware, they must be among those who are "the sufficiently intrepid" with respect to self-awareness. To deal with this simple self-mentoring, approaches using cognitive and psychodynamic psychology are provided here for consideration.

Uniqueness and Self-Knowledge

No matter what approach is used to understand stress—be it weighted in the direction of environment or personality—the individual is always a factor. This is observable in persons who come in for psychiatric or psychological treatment. I have found the following:

> . . . a significant turning point in therapy or counseling arrives when the individual seeking help is able to grasp the following, simple, seemingly paradoxical reality: When we truly accept our limits, the opportunity for personal growth and development is almost limitless. Prior to achieving this insight, energy is wasted on running away from the self, or running to another image of self.[12]

Such obviously is the case with most of us.

This should not be surprising. Poets, theologians, and great scientists have joined those in the mental health field to warn people to not be unconsciously pulled into trying to be someone you are not. In the words of e.e. cummings, for example, "To be nobody but yourself in a world which is doing its best, night and day, to make you everybody else—means to fight the hardest battle which any human being can fight, and never stop fighting."[13] Jewish theologian Martin Buber (1966) echoed this same theme from a slightly different angle by noting the following story to illustrate it:

> The Rabbi Zusya said a short time before his death, "In the world to come, I shall not be asked, 'Why were you not Moses?' Instead, I shall be asked, 'Why were you not Zusya?'"[14]

The point being made is that it can be a great struggle to be "simply ourselves"—especially when we are in a transferential role such as physician, nurse, or health specialist where people are turning to us when they are vulnerable much in the way they turned to parents and significant figures from the past. This cannot be prevented, but in terms of our own sense of self, we must be aware that this perception is based on their needs and personality and not on our abilities or objective reality. Being "extraordinary" is not being a superperson as some (including, unfortunately, some of our colleagues) want us to believe. Instead, it is being self-aware and in tune with the way our talents and the needs of those with whom we work in health care act in synchronicity. Accomplished inventor and global citizen R. Buckminster Fuller phrased it this way in terms of his own life and the dangerous lures he met during his life:

> The only important thing about me is that I am an average healthy human being. All the things I've been able to do, any human being, or anyone, or you, could do equally or better. I was able to accomplish what I did by refusing to be hooked on a game of life that had nothing to do with the way the universe was going. I was just a throwaway who was willing to commit myself to what needed to be done.[15]

Having a view such as that of Fuller takes a degree of humility. Yet, with such humility, not only do health care professionals avoid the unnecessary stress that comes from living as if the transferences put on them by patients are in fact a reality, but also the students whom seasoned practitioners are called to guide are helped. As Pfifferling, in a discussion of medical education, rightly indicates,

> Students can be exposed to the mistakes made by their faculty so that error in problem solving can improve learner behavior. Faculty self-disclosing behavior and modeling of personal/ professional humility to a student reinforce the necessity to be on guard against medical arrogance that can cost a patient his life. By self-disclosing mistakes to their students, the faculty prevent the student from becoming too arrogant or too distanced from the troubles of their patients, and provider/patient bonding is strengthened and improved.[16]

Humility and its connection with emotional sensitivity on the part of a physician, nurse, or allied health professional therefore are not signs of weakness. Instead, humility is a sign of balance, self-awareness, and maturity that raises the quality of interactions between patient and caregiver. For instance, as Coombs and Fawzy recognize, when medical education emphasizes only the "hands" (technique) and the "head" (knowledge) and fails to explore the role of the "heart" (emotional sensitivity), which in my mind includes an acceptance of one's failures, it diminishes not only the quality of the physician's own life but also the quality of patient care and mentoring of new interns and residents.[17]

To illustrate the potentially negative results that occur when the education of the heart is neglected, Coombs and Fawzy quote Donald Arnstein, who warns that such people will "live most of their emotional lives as children, taking seriously what deserves a smile, laughing at what deserves respect, and floating on the surface of experience, the depth of which is hidden to them" (story told by J. Mason in 1979 in forum lecture at Brigham Young University).[18]

Full self-awareness that includes such an awareness of our emotional sensitivity or lack of it is very elusive. In the words of poet Henry David Thoreau, "It is as hard to see oneself as to look backwards without turning round."[19] Yet, every effort must be made to increase self-understanding—not just to curb our errors but also to increase our self-respect because as Leech aptly notes, "You do not want to know someone whom you despise, even if, especially if, that someone is you."[20] One feeds the other and forms a positive circle. Self-respect is really true self-awareness.

To become clearer about ourselves, there is a need to expend energy, but it obviously helps to know the most productive and efficient way to do this. To best accomplish a sense of clarity about our feelings, beliefs, and actions, appreciating the value of discipline, noting inconsistencies and exaggerated emotions, and avoiding vagueness (a sign that the defense of unconscious repression is at work) would be helpful.

Embarking on a Disciplined Search

Self-awareness is an ongoing, dynamic undertaking that requires daily attention. When we have such a process in place, we can become more attuned to the rhythm of our personality and have our "psychological fingers" on the pulse of where we are emotionally with respect to an issue, a person, a challenge, or the general thrust of where our life is moving.

To accomplish this, we need to be aware of the ebb and flow of our reactions so we can become more sensitive to the subtle inconsistencies in our affect (i.e., experiences of sadness, depression, happiness, etc.), cognitions (ways of thinking, perceiving, and understanding), and actions. This provides us with a link to some of the motivations and mental agendas that lie just beyond our awareness—what some would refer to as our "preconscious." To be in a position for such an appreciation of ourselves, time must be taken to identify anything in the way we live that is incongruent so we can seek to understand the reason for the difference.

Instead, what often happens when we do, think, or feel something that is generally out of character for us is that we dismiss it as irrelevant or excuse it ("I was just tired, that is all"). However, when we do this and do not seek to accomplish a creative synthesis in understanding all parts of ourselves, we miss the normally buried treasures in our psyche that provide clues to material that is generally not available to us for consideration.

Elements of Clarity

One of the constants present when health care professionals seek help to avoid or limit the sources and symptoms of secondary stress is the temporary lack of clarity they are experiencing. In mentoring, the goal is to help them to clarify, to discern different approaches, and to problem solve, to find solutions to their inner and external stresses. To accomplish this, time must be taken to focus on the specifics of their reactions. This helps the person to move through conscious (suppression) and unconscious/preconscious (repression) avoidance or forgetting. By limiting vagueness and a tendency to generalize or gloss over details and feelings, information that lies just beyond our sense of awareness becomes available. So, rather than turning away from the seemingly unacceptable feelings, cognitions, impulses, and reactions, we face the anxieties that they produce as a price for learning more about ourselves. The benefit, of course, is greater self-knowledge and, in turn, more personal freedom. Rather than being limited by our blind spots in self-awareness and the waste of energy on defensiveness, by focusing on our interactions during the day we seek to become sensitive to *all* of our reactions—even the seemingly incongruous ones—as a way to deepen our knowledge.

The reason people resist clarity in life is that it cannot be limited to how others (e.g., patients, their families, or our colleagues) are stymied in denial. We also must look at our *own* behavior, cognitions, and affect. Clarity is a process by which we must be willing to look at how we are denying, minimizing, rationalizing, or hiding things from ourselves. Although we often say that we want to see ourselves and our situation as they truly are, conflict often arises when this happens because the responsibility then falls on us to

- Be aware of all of our own agendas—including the immature ones
- See our defensiveness and our tendencies to project blame onto others
- Find appropriate levels of intimacy with those with whom we interact
- Know how to deal with anger and the unhelpful reactions to failure
- Achieve a level of skill as a critical thinker

Awareness of Our Agendas

Thinking that we do things for one reason is naïve. In most cases, there are a number of reasons—some immature, some mature—that we do things. Because the reasons we do not like to acknowledge often remain beyond our awareness, clarity calls us to embrace all of them. In this way, the immature reasons can atrophy and the mature ones can grow and deepen. However, to accomplish this goal, we must first accept that we are all defensive in some unique way. Such an admission is an excellent first beginning because it does not put us in the position of asking, "Are we or aren't we?" Instead, it moves it out of the black-and-white situation to the gray areas where most of us live psychologically. When we look at all of the reasons why we reacted to a situation in the way we did, we can begin to appreciate why people react to us in the way that they do. Otherwise, we remain puzzled, feel misunderstood, and project all of the blame outward so as never to learn what are the dynamics and how to unravel them in any given situation.

For instance, if colleagues do not like to work with us in stressful situations, it would be helpful for us to know our part in it so we can work on decreasing the incidence of it. Once a candidate applying for a position as my assistant asked me, "Do you know how human resources is billing the main challenge of working with you?" Surprised—after all, how could there be *any* challenge in working with me?—I responded, "No, I don't." To which she noted with a smile, "They are billing you as a perfectionist who gives vague instructions and gets upset when they are not followed exactly." Impatience, anger, and other reactions on our part do not increase efficiency when we are working with colleagues in a difficult health care emergency. Blaming our reactions solely on other people's incompetence provides very limited information for improving the situation by changing our own behavior. Even if the others were not as prepared as they should have been to handle the medical emergency, reacting emotionally in a way that makes the situation deteriorate further certainly does not improve things.

Clarity calls us to recognize our agendas, face our own fears, understand the games we play with others, lessen our defensiveness, develop new coping skills, and create alternative ways to deal with stressful situations. Yet, to do this, we have to be honest. We also have to appreciate that this can have a positive domino effect in our life as a way of moving through the resistances we have to growth and change. When we start focusing on understanding individual interactions, larger questions open up as to whether we are getting enough rest or leisure, the right balance of time alone and with good friends, and how and when we are setting limits in all aspects of our life. It is important to recognize that the self is a limited entity that can be depleted if we do not involve ourselves seriously in a process of self-care.

Appropriate Intimacy

Healthy intimacy with others is a wonderful antidote to unnecessary stress and an effective inoculation against the destructive impact of the necessary pressures of health care work. Unfortunately, when distancing from others or overinvolvement or inappropriate involvement with others occurs, it adds to our problems in work and at home.

In medical and nursing school, as well as in allied health programs, little is taught on the topic of "transference." Transference occurs when a person views someone in the present as if he or she were a significant person from the past. It is a normal phenomenon that we experience everyday. For instance, when we see a police officer, clergyperson, or someone in authority, we may have a response that has nothing to do with the individual person but has all to do with what they represent for us. Patients and coworkers will often transfer positive and negative feelings onto physicians, nurses, and other health care professionals. Being aware of this so as not to absorb the negative transferences or believe and act on the positive ones by violating boundaries is essential.

When one is doing the best that can be done for a patient or is trying to be as supportive as possible to a colleague, it is very hard to recognize negative transference for what it is, but it is important that we do so as not to react negatively in kind. When feeling under great stress at work and/or feeling underappreciated or misunderstood at home, there is also a danger that one would become inappropriately involved with a patient or colleague who is transferring their positive feelings from the past onto us because we are in a caregiving role at a time of great vulnerability and need for them.

Some deal with this not by trying to be aware of what is occurring and discussing it with a trusted senior colleague or mentor but instead by distancing themselves from patients and colleagues alike. Doing this can be dangerous to our welfare and the good of the patients and our colleagues on a number of levels. First, being very distant can lead to callousness. When this happens, we become impervious to the feelings and needs of others. Also, with respect to our colleagues, real nongenital intimate relationships help one to understand oneself and to open oneself to others in ways that foster mutual support and friendship. In turn, this provides a basis from which we can reach out to patients and colleagues in need.

Learning from Our Negative Emotions

Negative emotions are psychological red lights indicating that we are dealing with situations with which we are unhappy or uncomfortable. However, beyond this, it is helpful to more fully understand how coming into contact with people who are depressed, angry, sarcastic, or dismissive of us can affect us. Otherwise, we will respond negatively, passive aggressively, or with "chronic niceness" because of the misguided feeling that absorbing patient and colleague anger is part of our job description. As I have indicated elsewhere, such an attitude is both dangerous and unnecessary:

> This leads to ulcers, unnecessary stress, depression, and outbursts of anger when all the "swallowing" of anger becomes too much. Negative emotions are like alcohol; they can be used or abused.
>
> With respect to anger, it needs to be recognized and addressed directly. In addition, if one sees or experiences depression, it too must be named and the source of it questioned. Hiding, belittling, or running away from such emotions because they are unpalatable is only postponing the problem until it gets worse for the other person or the [caregivers] themselves.
>
> Many . . . say: "I just don't know how to deal with angry people." To face such a fear of others' anger or the inexperience one might have in dealing with it, two steps usually are of help to get one started in confronting it.
>
> The first step is imagery. To image oneself dealing with an angry person and to see oneself responding with a sense of poise is a good exercise to practice in the privacy of one's own room. Another useful step when one is holding back from expressing anger in a constructive way is to ask one-

Table 2-1   Questions Regarding Our Experiences of Anger

- In what ways did I make myself angry today? (Not the passive: "What made me angry?"
- With whom did I choose to be angry today? (Once again, not the passive: "Who made me angry?")
- As well as the apparent "reason" I was angry, what other reasons might there be that I became annoyed, angry, or as upset as I was in this particular situation?
- What was my style of dealing with my emotional reaction? Did I try to conceal, deny, or play it down?
- How do I normally spontaneously allow my anger to rise and come to the surface of my awareness? Did I do that this time in a way that was destructive? Was I overly concerned that people would dislike me—even if I expressed my anger in a constructive manner?
- Was I able to recognize my anger before it was expressed inappropriately ("shotgun fashion" which broadly attacked the person and tried to scare him but didn't focus on the problem)?
- Did I have a realistic recognition that even good communication around something I am unhappy about may not solve the problem? Was I able to take satisfaction in the fact that opening up a discussion about differences is a worthwhile endeavor in itself?

---

self: "What is the worst thing that can happen if I confront someone?"

[Surprisingly more often than you would think] . . . there is a deep fear that the person will beat us up physically. In those instances I say . . . "If this person is not bigger or tougher than you, it won't happen; if the person is, have someone outside the confrontation area to help you if need be."

We must face our deepest fears about rejection, being beaten up or having our image stained, so we can face the blackmail we have set up in our own belief system. This belief system has been developed over a period of time and needs to be addressed so we don't have to continue to run from others' actual or perceived negative emotions.[21]

By asking ourselves a number of questions, we can arrive at a better recognition of both direct and indirect expressions of anger. It is also possible through self-questioning (Table 2-1) that we will see our motivations, fears, and interpersonal style more clearly.

The more this is accomplished, the more we will be withdrawing our projections, taking control of our lives, and, in the process, reducing unnecessary stress.

Facing Failure in a Productive Way

A reality in health care is that the more you are involved with persons who are suffering, the more you are going to fail. So, you had better be able to put failure in perspective. There is a myth that if one is up on the literature, pays attention to the patient, and provides an accurate diagnosis and regimen of treatment, failure is impossible; this myth is very destructive to the spirit of the physician, nurse, or allied health professional. Failure is part and parcel of involvement. Given the many demands and the inability to be perfectly "on" all the time, failure will occur. People are going to die—unfortunately and eventually because of our errors. However, although this is inevitable when we are constantly dealing with sick people, failure can still provide helpful information that will limit future mistakes. Failure teaches us to

- Recognize the dangers of pride and the need for openness
- Consider ways to avoid errors in the future
- Change factors that increase the possibility of failure
- Experiment with new approaches
- Learn about ourselves
- Improve technique and collaborative style
- Be sensitive to early warning signs of mistakes
- Consider the impact of negligence
- Uncover areas where further education/supervision is required
- Appreciate unrealistic expectations
- Improve pacing in one's work
- Acknowledge personal/professional limitations so they can be corrected or improved and so we can be more aware of the limitations that must remain unaltered

If failure is carefully considered rather than just becoming a source of self-condemnation or an impetus to blame, deny, or distort the situation, future patients will benefit immeasurably from the process of examination on your part. However, to accomplish this, professionals in health care must seek to be critical thinkers.

Critical Thinking

Critical thinking helps us to more clearly understand situations, patients, colleagues, and our agendas, negative emotions, attitudes, motivations, talents, and growing edges. This not only helps us to have a greater grasp of reality but also stops the drain of psychological energy that is necessary to be defensive or to protect our image. Because critical thinking is not natural, although we may think it is for us, it takes discipline, a willingness to face the unpleasant, and a stamina that allows one not to become unduly frustrated when we do not achieve results as quickly as we prefer with respect to our insights and growth.

The types of questions we must be willing to ask ourselves as critical thinkers are as follows:

- Am I willing to avoid seeing things simply in black and white and to entertain the various aspects and ambiguity in life?
- Can I appreciate that the "answer" or diagnosis I now offer is always tentative?
- When I am in a discussion of a patient, clinical situation, or even my own role, talents, and growing edges as a professional and a person, am I able to entertain both the possible and the probable without undue discomfort?
- Do I need to come to a quick solution or to take one side of an issue because I lack the intellectual stamina that encourages an open mind?
- Am I so uncomfortable with personal rejection, a tarnished image, or failure that I capitulate when I disagree with others?
- Am I willing to "unlearn" what I have learned that is not useful anymore and to be open to new techniques and approaches?
- Do I realize I resist changes in obvious and less noticeable ways and that one of my goals is to see some of my emotions and extreme reactions as red flags that can often indicate that I may be holding on because of fear, stubbornness, or some other defensive reason?

The willingness to be a critical thinker and to face questions like those given not only takes motivation but also involves an appreciation of how resistant most of us usually are without even knowing it.

Appreciating and Overcoming Your Own Resistance to Change

Change—even when we are aware that we have problems that need to be confronted—sometimes seems so elusive. As Rodman in his classic work on becoming a psychotherapist, "Keeping Hope Alive," notes, "Every patient stared at long enough, listened to hard enough, yields up a child arrived at from somewhere else, caught up in a confused life, trying to do the right thing, whatever that might be, and doing the wrong thing instead."[22] However, this point does not only hold for persons seeking counseling and psychotherapy. Everyone needs to recognize one's resistances as well, yet even when motivated to do so, this is sometimes easier said than done.

As Thomas Merton, contemplative and author of the classic autobiographical work "The Seven Story Mountain," laments, "All day I have been uncomfortably aware of the wrong that is in me. The useless burden of pride I condemn myself to carry, and all that comes with carrying it. I know I deceive myself . . . but I cannot catch myself in the act. I do not see exactly where the deception lies."[23] As a result, it is essential to understand as much as we can about our own hesitancy to both uncover resistances and act effectively to address those areas we need to change. This is especially so if you are a health care professional for whom stress is so intense and working through resistances can literally be the difference between life and death, burnout or not, and living with meaning or drifting in quiet blunted despair.

The concept of "resistance" in helping patients who are experiencing emotional distress has changed over the years in a way that is helpful for any helping professional wishing to overcome their own barriers to personal and professional growth.

> In the early years of psychology, a client's resistance to change was often looked upon as solely a *motivational* problem. When a person did not succeed in changing, the counselor felt: "I did my job in pointing out your difficulties. In return, you didn't do yours!" The blame rested upon the one seeking change. The goal was to eliminate the resistances and get the person motivated again.
>
> Now, we recognize that when someone resists change and growth in their personal and professional lives they are not pur-

posely giving family, friends, coworkers and counselors a hard time. Instead, they are unconsciously providing a great deal of critical information on problematic areas of their life given their personality style, history, and current situation. This material then becomes a real source of new wisdom for psychological growth, professional advancement, and spiritual insight.

Though we still believe motivation is an essential key to making progress, we see that persons seeking change must also gain certain knowledge about themselves and act on it if they wish to advance. Or in a nutshell: *Motivation or positive thinking is good, but it is obviously not enough.*[24]

One of the reasons that motivation to change is not a sufficient condition for the alteration of one's attitude, cognition, and behavior is that we fear that the demands of change may be too costly. For instance, we would have to see our own role in the problems we are having and do something about it. In addition, we worry about how other people will react when we seek to move away from defensiveness or unhealthy competitiveness. The move toward health is surprisingly upsetting to those who are used to "the devil they know" with his or her defensive style. It might even challenge them to change, and they would be uncomfortable in dealing with this. Finally, seeing our own role in our problems does cause some negative reflection about the past and how much time we have wasted in behaving as we have. Despite such resistances to insight and growth, though, the "advantages" of staying the same are very costly and the freedom offered by insight and change is very great.

Still, by knowing that it is not easy to change, we must recognize that we are up against resistance. In respecting the tyranny of habit and secondary gain, we must take whatever measures we can to make our steps toward self-knowledge and personal/professional growth more realistic. Two ways we can do this is by increasing our sensitivity to our defensiveness and by taking what actions we can to outflank our resistances.

Increasing Sensitivity to Resistances to Change . . .
and Outflanking Them

When we seek to export the blame for problems in our life, it is referred to as "projection." This defensive style is manifested in many obvious and quiet ways, including denying our role in mistakes or failures, excusing our behavior, contextualizing our actions, absolving ourselves, rationalizing failures, and generally removing ourselves from the equation while focusing on the negative roles others have played.

Part of the reason we do this is that when we try to take responsibility for our own role in various unpalatable events, we go overboard. Instead of trying to understand what part we played so we can learn from this, we move from remorse about what we have done to shame about who we are. We can tell when this occurs because we start to condemn ourselves and become hypercritical of our behavior, overly perfectionistic, unrealistic in our comparison with others in the field, and overresponsible with respect to the impact we did and can have.

Instead, I encourage people to take a step back from the event, to try to frame the situation in an objective way by imagining it was someone else you were looking at, and to seek to become intrigued about your role. This helps to avoid overly blaming others, condemning yourself, or getting discouraged when results do not happen immediately. To further reduce the resistance to change, several caveats I offer to outflank the blocks to growth are as follows:

1. Anything discovered does not have to be changed immediately.
2. No area should be condemned—just neutrally observed as if it were happening to someone else.
3. No area should be defended—no one is criticizing or attacking, just observing where the energy is being spent.
4. Observations—even disturbing ones—should be embraced as a wonderful treasure trove of information.
5. After each period of observation, the areas of concern should be written down so some record is kept of discovery.[25]

With these provisions in mind, I then suggest that persons consider the following principle: "*Where there is energy (positive or negative) there is usually a grasping and/or fear.* When the smoke of a strong reaction is present, the fire of desire is also usually present and we need to know what it is. Otherwise, rather than our passions being good energy, they may be the product of unexamined attachments."[26] They then keep us connected to views and convictions that are covering or distorting the truth rather than leading us to it. Classic signs that we are holding on include arguing, not sharing all the information or motivations with persons with whom we discuss the event, complaining that change in certain areas is unrealistic, stonewalling persons through an icy silence or monopolizing the situation, feeling misunderstood or totally ignored, and other strong emotions or off-putting actions.

On the other hand, there are also classic signs that a person does value change, growth, and insight both professionally and personally. Some of these signs are

- An ability to let go
- Receptive to new lessons . . .
- Not self-righteous
- Intrigue with one's own emotional flashing lights
- Disgust with . . . the endless wheel of suffering that comes from grasping and bad habits
- Curious, not judgmental
- Values experience
- Recognizes danger of preferences which prevent experiencing new gifts in life
- Awake to present; is mindful
- Appreciates quiet meditation
- Generous and alive
- Learns, reflects, and applies wisdom to daily life
- Rests lightly in life[27]

In recognizing and overcoming resistances to growth and change then, we are able to appreciate that the most important person in improving our situation is ourselves. We accept this responsibility not with a spirit of self-condemnation or overresponsibility but with a sense of intrigue about the possibility within ourselves. We can see that at times we are emotional and opinionated. We see that blindness like this occurs because of fear and hesitation that may be partially rooted in our past but are certainly centered in a belief system that is tyrannical and often wrong. This results in a style of "self-talk" that comes as our friend and seems to support us but in the end undercuts both our ability to see things clearly and our ability to have solid self-esteem based on knowing what is good about ourselves and what our growing edges are with a sense of equanimity.

Improving Self-Talk

One of the main contributions of cognitive-behavioral psychological theory is its ability to help people better appreciate how one's beliefs (schemata) and cognitions (ways of thinking, perceiving, and understanding) can affect the way we feel and behave. Unfortunately, dysfunctional ways of perceiving ourselves and the world are both common and often left unchallenged. Such inattention is psychologically dangerous.

Psychiatrist David Burns, in his popular book *Feeling Good*, illustrates how people fall prey to cognitive errors that may lead to depression, an overall sense of discouragement, or both. Perfectionistic medical and nursing professionals are in particular danger of such irrational thinking if they are not aware of it. Among Burns categories are the following:

ALL OR NOTHING THINKING: You see things in black-and-white categories. If your performance falls short of perfect, you see yourself as a total failure . . .

OVERGENERALIZATION: You see a single negative event as a never-ending pattern of defeat . . .

MENTAL FILTER: You pick out a single negative detail and dwell on it exclusively so that your vision of all reality becomes darkened, like the drop of ink that discolors the entire beaker of water . . .

DISQUALIFY THE POSITIVE: You reject positive experiences by insisting that they "don't count" for some reason or other. In this way you can maintain a negative belief that is contradicted by your everyday experiences . . .

EMOTIONAL REASONING: You assume that your negative emotions necessarily reflect the way things are: "I feel it, therefore it must be true . . .

SHOULD STATEMENTS: You try to motivate yourself with should and shouldn'ts. . . . The emotional consequence is guilt. When you direct should statements toward others, you feel anger, frustration, and resentment . . .

PERSONALIZATION: You see yourself as the cause of some negative external event which in fact you were not primarily responsible for.[28]

For me, the core of the issue here is as follows:

Negative thinking is quite common. For some reason, all of us seem to give more credence to the negative than to the positive. We can hear numerous positive things but somehow allow a few negative things to discolor and disqualify the previously affirming feedback we received. Therefore, we need to (1) pick up and recognize our negative thinking so we can (2) link the negative thoughts we have to the depressive/anxious feeling we experience, so (3) the negative self-talk we have can be replaced with a more realistic thought or belief. It is in this way that we structure changing our negative thinking so our negative beliefs can eventually be modified as well.

We can always—and, unfortunately, frequently do—find a negative comparison to make when we are reflecting on our thoughts, actions, and motivations. . . . Making negative comparisons between our situations and those of others is never a problem. Maintaining perspective . . . is the difficulty!

We may say we already know this but can't seem to put it into practice. When I hear this statement I think of Mark Twain's comment: "The difference between the right word and the almost right word is the difference between lightning and the lightning bug." We may say we know it, but unless we can truly recognize and short-circuit the negativity that causes insecurity [and] increases defensiveness . . . then we really don't know it. . . .[29]

As Ranier Maria Rilke in *Letters to a Young Poet*, a classic work probably all of us read at some point in our undergraduate education, wrote

Only someone who is ready for everything, who excludes nothing, not even the most enigmatical, will live the relation to another as something alive and will himself draw exhaustively from his own existence. For if we think of this existence of the individual as a larger or smaller room, it appears evident that most people learn to know only one corner of their room, a place by the window, a strip of floor on which they will walk up and down. Thus they have a certain security. And yet what dangerous insecurity is so much more human which drives the prisoner in Poe's stories to feel out the shapes of their horrible dungeons and not be strangers to the unspeakable terror of their abode. We, however, are not prisoners. No traps

or snares are set about us, and there is nothing which should
intimidate or worry us . . . We have no reason to mistrust our
world, for it is not against us. Has it terrors, they are *our* terrors;
has it abysses, those abysses belong to us; are dangers at hand,
we must try to love them.[30]

The issue once again is that the way we perceive something is just as
relevant as what we perceive. When we realize this, then we can see
that both successes and failures can be used to increase self-understanding and self-appreciation. This is so much more life giving than having
them only be the source of a constant see-saw of ups and downs in life
and in our work. When we recognize this, how we look at or question
ourselves changes dramatically, as does our overall results.

Questions to Ask in Interviewing Yourself

Self-understanding, not self-indictment, is at the basis of the self-questioning process. This is important to reflect upon again and again—especially when you are conducting a systematic self-evaluation of yourself,
your stresses, and the personal and professional goals you have. In addition to having this nonjudgmental attitude when interviewing yourself,
a *structured* approach might be helpful so that areas are not avoided or
missed. When we interview ourselves in an effort to uncover cognitive
and affectual styles, the chances are great that we may miss or unconsciously avoid some area. Therefore, to aid physicians, nurses, and allied
health professionals in the discerning process of improving self-awareness, a "Medical/Nursing Professional Secondary Stress Self-Awareness
Questionnaire" is provided (Table 2-2).

A questionnaire of this type has no right or wrong answers.
Although some might be surprised, there is a tendency to feel awkward or threatened by certain questions despite the fact that it is being
filled out in confidence for yourself. Writing the first thing that comes
to mind and trying to be exploratory—rather than judgmental—with
yourself help to avoid unnecessary defensiveness or the oppression some
of us have from within due to an archaic superego.

If a questionnaire of this type can elicit an almost matter-of-fact
style of answering, it will provide a wonderful resource of information
on how we are thinking, feeling, and acting in our professional and

Table 2-2 Medical/Nursing Professional Secondary Stress
Self-Awareness Questionnaire

Instructions: Find a quiet, comfortable, and private place. Read each question and respond on a separate sheet of paper by writing the first thing that comes to mind. Once you have completed a page, do not turn back to it or refer to it when working on the other pages. Work as quickly as you can without setting a pace that is too stressful.

1. What is the reason you believe denial is so prevalent in the medical setting with respect to stress for physicians, nurses, and allied health personnel? What are the most common lies you tell yourself about your own stress?
2. At this point, what are the most realistic and helpful steps you can take to prevent, limit, and learn from stress?
3. What are the ways you have heard that are excellent approaches to reducing stress and improving self-care but you feel are unrealistic in your case? What would it take to make them realistic? ("A miracle!" is not an acceptable answer.)
4. When you think of the terms "burnout," "compassion fatigue," and "chronic secondary stress," what do you think of in terms of your own life?
5. What are the issues that make you most anxious? What are the ones you deal with the best?
6. What are the types of situations or interactions from the past that still haunt you?
7. Given the realistic demands of work and family, what would it take to balance these two areas in your life a bit more? (List only those steps that can be realistically taken by you within the next 2 to 3 years.)
8. In your own case, what helps you to fall prey to the common masochistic tenet: The only worthy medical or nursing professional is the one involved enough to be on the edge of burnout or physical fatigue.
9. In what ways did your professional schooling, clinical rotations, modeling by supervisors, and initial work after graduation inadvertently teach you that taking care of yourself is a sign of weakness and that an unhealthy lifestyle is the price of being in the field of health care?
10. What are the "bad habits" of the people you observe in your profession that you do not want to emulate? How are you seeking to embrace the wonder, passion, and intense involvement in medicine and nursing without also absorbing the pathological side of the profession?
11. When you are under a great deal of stress, what fantasies do you have? What do you think are healthy fantasies you should act upon some day? What are the unhealthy ones that, if acted upon, would cause you and others harm?
12. What elements that are currently in your self-care protocol have been most beneficial for you? What are the least?
13. What do you struggle with most in your efforts to take care of yourself? Because your presence as a professional in the health care field means that de facto you are a bright and accomplished person, you would not think that these struggles should be so hard for you; why are they?

(Continued)

Table 2-2 (*Continued*)

14. How would people describe your attitudes toward work?
15. What should be included in your list of personal doubts and insecurities that most people would be surprised to know about you?
16. In health care, focus on the person and clinical situation that are before you is essential; what do you find are the main sources of external distraction and inner preoccupation that prevent you from doing this?
17. What are the most positive and negative affects your personality style has on the way you interact with patients? With staff?
18. When under extreme stress, what is the style of interacting with others and handling the situation that you would most like to change? What steps are necessary to produce such a change?
19. What would you include in your list of motivations for originally becoming a physician, nurse, or allied health professional? (Make the list as long as you can. Be sure to include any reasons you might now perceive as unrealistic or possibly immature—e.g., status, power over other people's life and death struggles, financial security, voyeurism, etc.—so you have as complete an accounting as possible.)
20. Has the primacy of certain motivations changed for you over time? If so, how? Why do you think this is so? If this is problematic in some way, what might you do about it? For those beneficial changes in priorities, how are you ensuring that they remain in focus for you?
21. What are the most awkward subjects for you to discuss in relationship to your emotional and physical well-being as a health professional?
22. Where do you feel your narcissism comes into play in your role in health care?
23. What would be included in a list of what you like best about being a physician, nurse, or allied health professional? What would be on the list of what you like least?
24. What is most surprising to you about the professional life you now have?
25. What are the most frustrating aspects of your professional life? Your personal life?
26. If you have ever considered changing specialties, moving to a different health care setting, or leaving the field, what are the reasons for this?
27. When you think of the profession you are now in, how would you describe it for someone thinking of entering the field now? Suppose someone asked you how you thought it would be different in 5 years, what would you say?
28. What are the most important self-care procedures you have put into place in the past 5 years? What has been their impact on you? What ways would you now like to modify your plan?
29. Given your own personality style, what types of patients do you find most challenging? What types of colleagues, subordinates, and supervisors are able to easily elicit an emotional reaction from you? Given this, what ways have you found to most effectively interact with them? (Praying for their early happy death is not a sufficient response.)
30. How would you describe the seemingly beneficial and adverse impacts your professional life has had on your personal life and vice versa?

31. What are the 5 mistakes that you fear most in your work?

32. What stresses do you think you can lessen in your life by giving them some attention? What stresses do you feel powerless to alter?

33. How would you describe the differences in the sources of stress and the approaches to self-care between other human services fields and that of medicine, nursing, and allied health?

34. How self-aware do you feel you are? On what do you base this conclusion? What would help you gain greater self-awareness?

35. If you were to divide your personal needs for happiness into "necessary" and "desirable," what would be on each list? What would be on similar lists ("necessary" and "desirable") for professional satisfaction and growth?

36. What information about yourself do you think you most like to hide even from yourself because it makes you uncomfortable to be aware of it?

37. What is your style of dealing with conflict? How would you improve your approach? To accomplish this, what is the next step you think you should take?

38. How much time alone do you need to remain balanced? What are the ways you see that such time is scheduled for yourself?

39. How do you know when you have lost your sense of perspective? What steps do you take to regain or maintain it?

40. What role does a sense of humor and laughter play in keeping yourself and the situation you are in from getting unnecessarily "heavy?"

41. What "little things" in life do you treasure and would miss if they were not present in your life? What are the big things? How do you show that you appreciate them?

42. Of what professional accomplishments are you very proud? What are some future ones you would very much like to achieve?

43. Describe how you organize your schedule and how much control you have in your life? Are there ways this might be improved?

44. When and with whom are you most apt to react in an angry way? In a cowardly way? By withdrawing? Through avoidance?

45. Would you and others at work and home best describe you as assertive, passive, passive-aggressive, or aggressive? Is there a difference between your style in your personal life and that in your professional life? If so, how would you account for that?

46. What are the major areas of imbalance in your life? How are you addressing them? If you are not, what are some of the reasons you feel it is important to do so at this point in your life?

47. Do you know how to observe your feelings and behavior and then seek to see what cognitions (ways of thinking, perceiving, and understanding) and beliefs (schemata) are giving rise to them? If so, do you then dispute your dysfunctional thoughts as a way to keep perspective and avoid unnecessary stress/depressive thinking/self-condemnation? If not, how might you improve this area of self-awareness, self-monitoring, and increased recognition of the style of one's self-talk, especially when under undue stress or after a failure?

(Continued)

Table 2-2 (*Continued*)

48. What are the most unhealthy ways you are now meeting your needs or "medi-cating" yourself? What unhealthy gratifications are you concerned that you might avail yourself of in the future? What are you doing to prevent, limit, or avoid this from happening?

49. What is the overall design of your daily, weekly, monthly, and yearly breaks for leisure, relaxation, quiet, and recreation? How would you describe your feelings about these times (e.g., guilt, "I deserve it," feeling uncomfortable, preoccupied with cases, blissful, resentment that they are too few and far between, etc.)?

50. What are the types of negative statements you normally make to yourself when you fail?

51. What are the healthiest ways you cope with life's difficulties? What are the most immature and unhealthy ways?

52. In what ways are you collaborative with other members of the health care team? What are the benefits and struggles you experience with such collaboration?

53. What professional and personal resentments do you still carry, and when are they most likely to surface?

54. Have you had any significant losses in the past several years? If so, what has your reaction been to them—initially, recently, now?

55. How do you view yourself in terms of physical aspects of your life (e.g., attractiveness, physical health, eating/drinking/weight/smoking/medication and illegal drug use, and exercise patterns)?

56. What is your reaction to the statement, "Much of medical care is still an art rather than an exact science"?

57. What are your feelings about asking for help in your personal life from your family? A colleague? Professional organization? One's physician? A psychiatrist, psychologist, or counselor? A clergyperson?

58. In your professional life, when have you been tempted to step over personal, sexual, financial, or other appropriate boundaries you should have with your patients or colleagues?

59. Is there someone in your circle of friends who is both kind yet clear and direct with you, so you would feel at ease to share anything but also would feel you are getting honest guidance?

60. In what clinical situations or with what type of clients do you feel most emotionally vulnerable? In other words, when have you reacted by going to either the extreme of overinvolvement or preoccupation or by closing down emotionally and seeing them as simply "a case," "bed 2 in room 342," or "the gallbladder in intensive care"?

personal lives. The combination of answers can also provide themes that offer a springboard to real understanding and insight into our personalities. Of course, on the other hand, those individuals who are defensive and try to coach their answers or are vague will end up with little helpful material other than the conclusion that how they look to themselves without reflection is the same after time is spent reviewing their intrapersonal and interpersonal styles, talents, growing edges, and personal/professional hopes and goals.

In addition to being a guide to quiet reflection by yourself, the responses to a questionnaire can be helpful in speaking with a mentor, trusted family member or coworker, or counselor or as material for a discussion group. Another value in its use is that it provides a record for us. By having in writing a clear description of our thoughts and feelings about key areas in our lives, we can go back to them again and again to see how they match our current outlook. Moreover, once we have our original impressions down on paper, our unconscious censoring mind cannot change what we have written and our memory cannot distort our impressions as easily. A final advantage in taking out the time is that by reviewing previously noted reactions, we can discover what additional thoughts we have now about such issues. By doing this, we can tap into our personal wisdom and expand upon it.

As in any challenging undertaking, there are resistances to taking the time to accomplish the task at hand. Yet, if someone early in your education told you that you would improve your chances significantly to get into medical or nursing school or into a graduate school of allied health by taking only an hour or so of your time to complete a questionnaire, you would probably jump at it. The same can be said of completing this questionnaire with respect to the remaining years of your professional career. By taking time to focus on yourself in a helpful, guided way, there is immeasurable aggravation you can avoid and pleasure, control, and balance in your life you can enjoy.

Reviewing Your Responses

Once a questionnaire of this type is completed, it is sometimes helpful in your reflective process and in discussion of the topics with trusted others to have a guide. However, even before you consider a series of suggestions on what a particular question might elicit in terms of responses, the point should be made that great caution is necessary in attempting to consider what you have written. Interpretations or attempts to more deeply understand your responses should always be seen as tentative. Even the most experienced psychologists or psychiatrists can make incorrect or partially correct interpretations or explanations of individual responses. Therefore, a form such as the "Medical/Nursing Professional Secondary Stress Self-Awareness Questionnaire," once again, is meant as a springboard for further reflection on your part or discussion with someone else as to what your response might mean if expanded upon or taken to its logical conclusion in terms of implications for self-care, self-knowledge, or the prevention or limitation of secondary stress in your life. Remember: The knowledge provided by your responses to this form is to help you obtain an even better understanding than you have now of your lifestyle patterns, talents, and growing edges. The questionnaire is not an exercise in guilt enhancement or to increase your narcissism. Attitude toward the review will be the major factor in gleaning valuable information from it. Finally, in reviewing what you have written, there are two final points to consider:

1. Before beginning the review, try to set the stage for a nonjudgmental review of the material by emphasizing the need to have a sense of intrigue rather than defensive projection, self-condemnation, or discouragement. One way to accomplish this is to imagine that you are looking at the profile of someone else rather than yourself. Such an artificial distancing from the material might help in limiting judgmental or unduly defensive tendencies.

2. Read each response to each individual question and think about the meaning of what you have written. The pace of this process will depend on each individual. Sometimes we spend a good deal of time on a particular response that touches a personal chord in our lives at the time. Other times, the area being questioned has little emotional weight or application at this time in your life.

Having offered these provisos, a listing of *some* factors that may be helpful to consider in reflecting on your responses to each of the questions is provided (Table 2-3). Just use them as a catalyst to your own ideas. In this way, you will make the evaluation of the form your own and, with greater self-knowledge, be more apt to follow through on what you

Table 2-3 Individual Question Reflection Guide for the Medical/Nursing
Professional Secondary Stress Self-Awareness Questionnaire

1. We often tell ourselves "lies" about our behavior and make excuses for it
   because we do not want to give up the secondary gain involved or expend the
   effort needed to decrease the amount of stress we are under. Until the "payoffs"
   we receive for the behavior are unmasked as too costly and unnecessary, even
   the most destructive and immature defensive behavior will remain to cause us
   stress.
2. "Realistic" and "helpful" are important words in this question because they try
   to help us get around the resistance to change that is present when we feel any
   steps to reduce stress in health care are beyond us; therefore, we do not have to
   do anything.
3. This question seeks to push us a bit further in an effort to get us to be more
   assertive and creative in our planning and actions regarding the stress in life.
4. Too often we resist change by being global in our definitions of what is caus-
   ing stress in our lives. This question seeks to get more specific causes out in the
   open so they can be addressed more directly either by ourselves or with our
   mentor/peer group.
5. This question allows us to make an inventory of our strengths and areas of
   vulnerability or growing edges. The longer and more detailed the two lists, the
   more useful will be the responses. Also, looking for patterns in the list can be
   helpful in terms of planning interventions or attitude/schedule changes.
6. The only memory that is a problem is the one intentionally forgotten or
   unconsciously repressed because it retains power without our being aware of
   it. This question gives an opportunity to be honest again regarding those past
   events that are still sapping energy from us now and unconsciously impact-
   ing our behaviors in the present. PTSD includes such memories, but anyone
   who works in health care, by nature of their work, have experienced traumatic
   occurrences and need to have a clear awareness of them—not in order to blame
   oneself but to learn from them.
7. In health care, there is a general tendency toward an imbalance in favor of work
   over one's personal life. This question provides an opportunity to take initial
   steps to change this imbalance a bit. One of the goals in phrasing the question
   again with the word "realistic" is to try to break the logjam that occurs when we
   feel overwhelmed and think nothing can be done. Perspective and attitude have
   tremendous power; although people who burn out often lose an awareness of
   this and feel that unless someone else changes my environment, little of benefit
   can result.
8. Once we accept the mantle of "only a burned out professional really cares and
   works hard," the psychological cost is immense. Moving against this societal and
   professional myth is essential if one is to undertake a program of self-care.
9. This is an opportunity to divide the people who we thought were professionally
   competent and personally attractive from the dysfunctional behavior they may
   have also modeled.

(Continued)

Table 2-3 (*Continued*)

10. As a follow-up to question 9, this one asks for more information on how we can carry on the good heritage of our role models and leave their parallel defensive sides so we can become more healthy in how we carry out medical/nursing roles.

11. There are some fantasies we should act on and others that would be dangerous if we did. Knowing the difference *ahead of time* is essential, so acting out or violating boundaries with colleagues or patients is never done with the rationalization after the fact that "It just happened."

12. This raises the need to have a self-care protocol and starts us to think in a more-focused manner about the helpful and destructive ways one deals with the pressures in one's personal and professional life.

13. This question is designed to have one face their own resistances and defenses with the same energy and intellectual stamina as other issues are faced in life.

14. "Workaholism" is a pattern that seems to go unchecked in many a health care professional's life; this question helps one not to gloss over the work style that everyone seems to acknowledge is present in us but that we cannot seem to fully grasp ourselves. People continue to endure an immense amount of unnecessary stress with either the response "It's part of the territory of being a nurse (doctor, allied health professional)" or "That's just the way I am."

15. This allows us to take a step back and to acknowledge the human doubts and insecurities that all people have. This is important because much defensive or compensatory behavior is driven by such unexamined dynamics.

16. Distractions waste a tremendous amount of time in health care. Mistakes are often attributed to a lack of attention. This question helps us to see how we might systemically avoid unnecessary distraction or understand the dynamics involved in what needlessly preoccupies us at times when at work.

17. Making a list of how our personality both negatively and positively affects certain types of individuals or all people when we are in certain moods equips us to better use our style of dealing with the world. By having greater awareness in this area, we can avoid so many potential relational problems that it is worth returning to this question to see what else we might add as illustrations of when and how we improved or made situations worse. It is very hard to do this because of the tendency to project the blame onto a patient or staff member on the one hand or simply blame ourselves on the other. Clarity and a nonjudgmental approach to ourselves and our behavior are needed here.

18. Knowing your own stress points and when you are particularly vulnerable is essential. Even basic steps like knowing when to keep quiet until we understand why we are reacting so strongly and can regain more of our composure can make a major difference in the stress level of interactions with others.

19. In many cases we believe we know why we entered the field of medicine, nursing, or allied health. However, there were many overlapping mature and immature reasons that we probably have not thought about. Having this information is very valuable so that we can appreciate how to let the mature reasons grow and the other ones atrophy or take their proper place rather than ascending to a level where we make decisions for the wrong reasons.

20. Revisiting motivations that inspired and challenged us is essential if we are to keep and deepen the roles we have assumed in the lives of others. This reflection is very important, especially with the jaded views of many in the culture with respect to health care and the possible beneficial roles they might play in it.

21. There are many awkward subjects that are sensitive for us to discuss with others that we do not reflect on "in safety" with ourselves. This question gives us permission and encouragement to take some time to look at what we are sensitive about and to start asking ourselves what we can do about it.

22. Healthy narcissism is good. It encourages us to take credit for good work and to be happy that we are in key roles caring for others and helps us recognize when we become defensive because our ego is getting in the way when it should not.

23. This question reacquaints us with both the joy and pain of being in health care. It is being asked so that there is greater clarity about what we do not like to see and how it can be changed in some way; even minor alterations in a number of areas can provide great summative relief. But more than that, by getting more clear about what we like best, we can remember to enjoy and take strength from these areas when they are encountered each day.

24. This is a standard "taking stock" question that asks us what is going on that we did not anticipate so that if we need to do something about it we can do it before we become too derailed personally and professionally.

25. Frustrations drain energy. By naming them we are taking the first step to understanding why they are so frustrating to us whereas others do not find them to be so. Once they can be understood in this way, they will lose some of their power; then we can catch ourselves when we repeat this pattern so we do not continue it any longer than need be.

26. Thoughts of job change often come during times when we have an aggregate of negative elements in our professional lives. By reviewing when and how we thought of moving or actually did, we can learn from this process in ways that prevent unnecessary moves or help us realize better when such a significant change is needed to relieve intractable stress or open up new possibilities.

27. This question is important for all of us to ask so we can be honest with ourselves as to how we feel about the field and our role in it. It also pulls us into the future to give some sense of the tone of our outlook, and it begs the question, What would I need to do to make this more positive for myself?

28. Our self-care protocol is examined here. At the very least, this question will encourage us to see if we have a plan in place. If it is informal, then it will help us write down what we are actually doing and give us a sense of how we might improve it.

29. Knowing who is able to "push our emotional buttons" is an important antidote to unnecessary stress. This question revisits this area so greater clarity, which is much needed on this topic if we are to remain psychologically healthy in tense situations, can be gained. Otherwise, the only thing that will happen is that we will project the blame onto certain types of people or blame ourselves for losing our temper or acting out.

(Continued)

Table 2-3 (*Continued*)

30. Looking at the interchange between personal and professional well-being and how they affect each other helps us see that most adversity involves a more complex dynamic than we at first imagined it to have.

31. Breaking down fear into specifics allows us to discuss them with mentors and colleagues who we trust, so we can deal with the fears constructively rather than having them haunt us to no purpose. Just a naming and discussion of them can help alleviate stress in this area.

32. Powerlessness is an element in all of us. However, once again, perception and attention to such areas tend to diminish those areas that heretofore have been ignored and allowed to have control because of a lack of examination.

33. This is a chance to see what, if any, differences we feel about our profession and the stresses it holds as opposed to other fields. It allows us also to normalize some of our stress because we have much in common with persons in many fields but do not often acknowledge this.

34. Methods that lead to self-awareness such as reflection, meditation, journaling, receiving and giving supervision, personal daily debriefing, receiving mentoring, and formal/informal peer group discussions can help us become better attuned to our styles. This question helps us visit this area to see if any or all of these approaches are present in some way, and if not, why not.

35. By breaking down needs, we can begin to see those cases where we are depriving ourselves of essential needs for personal or professional well-being and where we have developed a series of induced needs that are psychologically costing us too much.

36. This question again visits the issue of shame. It allows us to free up those areas we have partially hidden even from ourselves so we can finally learn more from them and let them take a more appropriate place in our psyche rather than dominating it from within.

37. Each person has a different style of dealing with conflict. It is not good or bad; it just "is." By taking this approach and seeking to see the pros and cons of our style, we can take steps to improve upon it. Most people focus on whether the other person is right or wrong rather than on the style of conflict resolution. That is why this question, if responded to in detail, can be very fruitful and can be a significant factor in stress reduction for ourselves and for those with whom we interact.

38. Time alone is often considered a luxury or seems to just happen at times in our schedule. However, whether you are an introvert or an extrovert, time alone is psychologically needed for renewal, reflection, and reassessment and to break the movement of an often-driven schedule. Having greater intention on where, how, and when to insert periods of solitude is necessary for one's mental health and for those who are religiously minded is an element of most major spiritualities.

39. Our loss of perspective is often more evident to others than to ourselves. However, there are signs that we have lost distance and a sense of proportion. They include extreme emotion, withdrawal, an unnecessary increase in the pace of activity, and preoccupation. Once we know this, we can then ask ourselves how

to best regain perspective. It may be by taking a few minutes alone on a short walk around the hospital or to the lavatory, a telephone call to a friend, or just remaining silent until we regain more of our composure. This approach helps us realize that each day we lose perspective and need to regain it in some way. It also prevents the three classic dangers that come about when perspective is lost: projection, self-blame, and discouragement. Intrigue with the dynamics within us and within the context in which the loss of perspective occurred is naturally more healthy and productive. Answering this question fully helps support this good movement in our professional and personal lives.

40. Too often, on the way to taking our work seriously, we take ourselves too seriously. This question highlights this reality for all of us and helps us remember to continually appreciate that laughter is good medicine and a sense of humor keeps things light whenever possible.

41. Deep gratefulness is one of the major preventatives and antidotes to a loss of perspective. We have much to be grateful for—including our roles in health care, which not everyone can or is willing to undertake. Gratefulness is not natural for most of us, whereas negative reactions seem to rise spontaneously and without effort. Self-training in this area, starting with greater awareness that all is a gift, can provide an immeasurable factor in the prevention of burnout. This is so because when you are feeling constantly nourished by your surroundings, you retain a better sense of balance—gratefulness increases our sensitivity to what events and people are giving us so we do not take them for granted, belittle them, or in fact miss them.

42. Taking stock of your accomplishments is an act of healthy narcissism. It also aids, once again, in prevention of the loss of perspective that comes when we just focus on the failures, absences, and struggles without seeing how far we have come. It also aids in planning for the future, which stirs up new hope in our hearts rather than having us just go through the motions every day.

43. Time management is often not taught in schools of nursing, medicine, or allied health. Yet, one of the causes of stress is disorganization or distraction at work. This question raises this issue to imply that there is more in our control than we are willing to acknowledge. In developing a self-care protocol, this area must be addressed in some way so we can use management/organizational skills to lessen stress. (This is addressed in Chapter Four on developing a self-care protocol, and further recommended readings in the area are also included there.)

44. By picturing actual people in our lives who cause attack-or-flight reactions, we can begin to better understand what it is that this type of person is triggering in our lives and so better deal with it. Once again, in most people's lives, the fact that certain people or personality types upset us is accepted as a given that cannot be changed. In medicine and nursing, this is a luxury of avoidance that must not be accepted, because we need to deal with such persons again and again.

45. Appreciating our style by honestly looking at ourselves should be easier at this point in the questionnaire because by now, we should be into the exercise of looking with a sense of intrigue and not with condemnation or denial. As we do this, it is important to begin to see the differences in our styles at work and

(Continued)

Table 2-3 (*Continued*)

at home and to try to better understand them. It will help in improving our interaction skills both at home and in our health care work setting.

46. Imbalances need not remain in our lives. They also need not be radically corrected overnight. Such a desire often ends up in our acting rashly rather than courageously to provide the necessary balance that will result in personal and professional well-being.

47. Picking up our feelings about things and then looking at what we are thinking and believing that may be dysfunctional and responding to them with thoughts that are more healthy are important steps in maintaining perspective and mental health. This question highlights this and helps us to raise the volume of our "self-talk" so we do not let negative thinking act as the invisible puppeteer in our psyche.

48. Work-a-holism, alcohol abuse, improper use of medication, sexual acting out, and compulsive activity (eating, buying, or gambling/stock market speculation) are just a few ways in which we "self-medicate." Knowing how, when, and to what extent we do this is an important first step in addressing this problematic area and is often one of the leading steps that we deny.

49. Taking time off during the day, week, month, and year is a conscious decision by those who effectively prevent and limit burnout. This area, as well as our feelings about them, is important to address as part of self-care.

50. Failure is part and parcel of involvement. The more we are involved and the more delicate problems we must face in health care, the more we will fail. That is a statistical reality because we cannot be perfect. Case closed. Therefore, knowing how we deal with failure, because it is often a part of what we do, would help diminish unnecessary anxiety and avoidable stress.

51. This question addresses overall style when we are faced with obstacles and asks for an inventory of our talents and defenses. As in some of the other questions, this seeks a review and also goes hand in hand with other questions to check the reliability of our previous responses.

52. Collaboration has often been seen as necessary but not realistic by many in health care. Yet, to be effective, health care needs to be a team effort in which each member of the team is respected, given as much autonomy as is appropriate, and has input into the health care program offered for the patient. An individual's understanding and attitude toward collaboration are explored in this question.

53. Resentments are psychological powder kegs that lie in the preconscious and may break through when triggered by an event or a person in our environment—especially when sleep deprivation or another problem/lack is present to make us more vulnerable. Unearthing these resentments so they do not remain as hidden psychological cancers that go unnoticed but continue to grow and devour us from within is obviously necessary.

54. Because dealing with the issues of death and dying is part of the territory for health care professionals, being aware of our own losses and how we have dealt with them or avoided dealing with them is quite helpful.

55. Taking note of our physical prowess and those elements that add or are destructive to it is something that is paradoxically avoided by many in health care. This

question asks for a detailed response that is undertaken without blame but with honesty and a willingness to consider measured change that will not be abandoned as in the case of a diet that leaves us permanently deprived.

56. Not every error in medical/nursing care is malpractice. No physician or nurse can be perfect in their diagnosis or intervention with all patients. This is a reality of the fact that medicine itself is not perfect. How we answer this question provides some insight into our view of the expectations we have of ourselves and the field.

57. We can never go it alone. Also, sometimes it is important to treat ourselves to a defined period of therapy or mentoring so we can work through failures, deepen our personal lives, and learn new creative ways of improving personal and professional well-being. This question looks at how we avail ourselves of help, collaboration, supervision, and support.

58. Honesty in this question allows us to pick up the "emotional flags" that will warn us when we might violate boundaries with a patient or colleague. Everyone has a vulnerable place in their lives where boundary violation is possible. Knowing ahead of time what these may be or what type of person with whom we would be most vulnerable is essential.

59. This question identifies those with whom we feel both freedom and clarity. At the very least, asking it points to the tenet that if we do not have a person like this, we run the risk of going off course in our professional and personal lives. It also points to the need to ensure we have steady contact with someone like this and, if we do not, to find someone who can fit this role.

60. Becoming callous or overemotional is a constant danger in health care. This question is designed to help us explore when and how this happens. As in the other questions in this questionnaire, it is asking us not to take our reactions for granted but to explore them further so we can both understand ourselves better and plan for change that is productive both professionally and personally.

think are the logical, realistic self-care steps you develop after review of the final two chapters in this book.

Objectives of Chapter Two

- Have a greater appreciation for the need to take time, on an ongoing basis, for reflection to see where and how we are losing perspective in life
- Be more sensitive to the fact that the positive and negative roles ascribed to health care professionals are not in fact real
- Know the definition of "transference" and the implications of persons reacting to health care professionals in ways that are

more in line with early life experiences for them than with the realistic personality and behavior of the nurses, physician, or allied health professional

- Be aware of the type of questions we can ask ourselves to gain a better recognition of the dynamics and both direct and indirect experiences and expressions of our anger
- Have a sense of the various ways failure can teach us
- Be familiar with the kinds of questions we must be willing to ask ourselves as critical thinkers
- Understand the concept of "resistance"
- Know David Burns' categories of irrational thinking and ways to address them
- Fathom the information on personal patterns in secondary stress that result from responding to a structured self-awareness questionnaire on this area

Additional Books to Consider

What Are You Feeling, Doctor? by J. Salinsky and P. Sacklin of the United Kingdom is a recent book published on identifying and avoiding defensive patterns in patient care. A general book on self-awareness that is a classic is Eric Berne's *Games People Play.* In addition, there are relevant sections in my two books *Riding the Dragon: 10 Lessons for Inner Strength in Challenging Times* and *Simple Changes: Quietly Overcoming Barriers to Personal and Professional Growth* that may prove useful.

Notes

1. L. Southgate, "Foreword," in J. Salinsky and P. Sacklin (Eds.), *What Are You Feeling, Doctor?* (Oxford, UK: Radcliffe Medical Press, 2000), viii.

2. E. Baker, *Caring for Ourselves* (Washington, DC: American Psychiatric Association, 2003), 15.

3. J. Coster and M. Schwebel, "Well-Functioning in Professional Psychologists," *Professional Psychology: Research and Practice*, 28 (1997): 10.

4. D. Block, "Foreword," in C. Schott and J. Hawk (Eds.), *Heal Thyself* (New York: Brunner/Mazel, 1986), ix.

5. *Ibid.*, ix.

6. R. Cole, quoted in R. Riegle, *Dorothy Day: Portraits by Those Who Knew Her* (Maryknoll, NY: Orbis, 2003), 140.

7. R. Wicks, *Touching the Holy* (Notre Dame, IN: AMP, 1992), 115.

8. A. Bloom, *Beginning to Pray* (Ramsey, NJ: Paulist Press, 1970), 39.

9. S. Suzuki, quoted in D. Chadwick, *The Crooked Cucumber* (New York: Broadway, 1999), 308.

10. Source unknown.

11. D. Brazier, *Zen Therapy* (New York: Wiley, 1995), 14.

12. R. Wicks, *Availability* (New York: Crossroad, 1986), 5, 6.

13. e. e. cummings, unpublished letter to a high school editor, 1955.

14. Martin Buber, *Way of Man* (New York: Lyle Stuart, 1966), Chapter 1.

15. R. Buckminster Fuller, quoted in R. Wicks, *Op. Cit.* (1986), 6.

16. J.-H. Pfifferling, "Cultural Antecedents Promoting Professional Impairment," in C. Scott and J. Hawk (Eds.), *Heal Thyself* (New York: Brunner/Mazel, 1986), 14.

17. R. Coombs and F. Fawzy, "The Impaired-Physician Syndrome: A Developmental Perspective," in C. Scott and J. Hawk (Eds.), *Heal Thyself* (New York: Brunner/Mazel, 1986), 55.

18. *Ibid.* 55.

19. Henry David Thoreau, quoted by W. H. Auden in "Introduction" in D. Hammarskjold, *Markings* (New York: Knopf, 1976), ix.

20. K. Leech (San Francisco, CA: Harper and Row, 1980), 43, 44.

21. R. Wicks, "The Stress of Spiritual Ministry: Practical Suggestions on Avoiding Unnecessary Distress," in R. Wicks (Ed.), *Handbook of Spirituality for Ministers, Vol. 1* (Mahwah, NJ: Paulist Press, 1995), 254–255.

22. R. Rodman, *Keeping Hope Alive* (New York: Harper and Row, 1985), 5.

23. Thomas Merton, *A Vow of Conversation* (New York: Farrar, Straus & Giroux, 1988), 161.

24. R. Wicks, *Simple Changes* (Notre Dame, IN: Thomas More/Sorin Books, 2000), 9.

25. *Ibid.*, 70–71.

26. *Ibid.*, 71.

27. *Ibid.*, 78, 79.

28. D. Burns, *Feeling Good* (New York: New American Library, 1980), 40–41.

29. R. Wicks, *Living Simply in an Anxious World* (Mahwah, NJ: Paulist Press, 1988), 30, 31.

30. R. Rilke, *Letters to a Young Poet*, revised edition translated by M. D. Herter Norton (New York: Norton, 1954), 68–69.

THREE

Drawing from the Well of Wisdom

Three Core Spiritual Approaches to Maintaining
Perspective and Strengthening the Inner *Life of the*
Physician, Nurse, and Allied Health Professional

Existential psychiatrist Irving Yalom once advised novice therapists to "Nurture the shudder; don't anesthetize the pain."[1] There is much to be learned in the darkness—especially if we have the psychological tools and spiritual wisdom to draw strength from these experiences.

In preparation for Grand Rounds with the Radiology Oncology Department at the University of Maryland, I interviewed a physician who was trying to develop a series of systemic approaches for preventing burnout in her staff. She was well aware that some of her technicians faced a unique danger when working with young patients, especially those with a poor prognosis. Because younger patients tend to visit and form relationships with those who provide their treatment more often than do older patients, the technicians are more apt to develop a personal rather than a professional concern for their welfare. When this happens and the young person dies, it sometimes has a psychologically devastating effect on the technicians who were responsible for their treatment.

Although the source of such stress cannot be prevented, the way it affects the medical professional does not have to be totally negative. As a matter of fact, even amid the suffering, maybe even *because* of it, when one has a sense of meaning in one's life, then a strong appreciation of both the welcome and unwelcome aspects of life and all it holds may become even deeper and more compassionate.

One physician who was working in Somalia during a devastating famine was approached by an interviewer for National Public Radio with the following question: "Doctor, how can you stand all of this? The old people are dropping like flies. And the children are dying in such numbers that you are stacking them up in the corner like firewood rather than burying them immediately? How can you stand it?" (You could hear the pain in his voice.) The physician stopped, turned to the interviewer, and said: "When you watch this horror on television in the U.S. you are overwhelmed, aren't you?" When the reporter from NPR nodded, the physician went on: "Well, we in country feel the same pain *but* there is one difference." The interviewer in an incredulous voice asked: "*What* difference?" And the physician softly responded: "You can't lose hope as long as you are making friends."

How nurses and medical practitioners *perceive* their work, the events that take place during the day, and the people they encounter along the way make all the difference. Due to this, an increasing number of health care professionals I have encountered now seem to use aspects of the wisdom literature of the major religions as a resource to maintain a sense of psychological perspective. The feeling seems to be that it would be as foolish to disregard this information as it would be to ignore new advances in medicine simply because we are unfamiliar with them.

For instance, a great deal has been recently published about the roles of faith and spirituality in a patient's healing process and attitude toward stress. Piedmont's recent work,[2] which bears this out, is based on the thesis that a person who has well-developed spirituality is more apt to have a positive outlook than is someone with a poorly developed one. And so, he believes that those with a highly developed spirituality are better equipped to cope with the psychological suffering and physical pain associated with illness or trauma. In addition, as Baker summarizes,[3]

> Empirical data tends to support the myriad personal testimonies about the relationship between spirituality and psychological and physical well being (W.R. Miller, 1999). Clinical research supports the effects of prayer, contemplation, meditation, yoga, and ritual in reducing medical symptoms and improving medical recoveries.[4,5] A renowned researcher of mind-body practices, Herbert Benson[6] speculated that spiritual experience serves as a physical balm to counter the rapid

pulse and adrenaline rush associated with stress. Other research reveals a relationship between elements of spirituality (e.g., connection with others and self, sense of meaning and purpose in life, hopefulness and optimism) and higher levels of psychological functioning (W.R. Miller, 1999).

Similar positive findings have been reported with respect to religion. Pargament, a respected researcher in this area, points out that "every religion offers a set of cognitive reframing mechanisms to help individuals conserve a sense of meaning in life in the face of what may seem to be senseless, unbearable or unjust."[6] At the very least, he notes that "coping strategies can take a special significance when cloaked in sacred garb." According to Hood and associates, religion also helps people regain a sense of control that helps them cope and adjust when they are faced with difficult situations.[7]

There still remains (in medicine especially) a caution or, at the very least, a hesitancy about discussing where this fits in the life of the physician, nurse, or allied health professional. This is understandable if we speak of religion with its canons; this is a very private area in everyone's life. One Orthodox Jewish dermatologist noted to me that he did not speak of his faith in front of those who worked for him. Yet, in many cases it was this very faith that gave his life meaning, structure, and purpose. Medicine was only one outgrowth of this. Moreover, he reported that stress in his life was lessened because of the sense of covenant he felt with God and the community of which he was a part. The ritual and rhythm of going to *shule* and the other aspects of the praxis of his faith gave him a structure and *raison d'être* that allowed his sense of perspective to flourish. The readings that he and other Jewish healing professionals absorb as part of their lives are, in some cases, the forerunners of the sound psychology we take for granted today.[8]

For instance, in the Jerusalem Talmud we read that when we die, we will be held responsible for all the gifts that we have been given that we did not enjoy. There is not just an emphasis on work and sacrifice but also a caution that we should not be "pyromaniacs of the soul." Life is to be enjoyed in its fullness—an important message for physicians, nurses, and allied health personnel prone to workaholism.

Beyond the Talmud, Jewish spiritual writers also warn against getting in over your head financially because of greed or the creeping growth of induced needs that can rule your life and create unnecessary stress.

Christian sacred scripture and spiritual literature also offer an awareness of the power that attitude and thinking play in life. The *New Testament*, for instance, proclaims, "If your eye is good, your whole body will be good." This is very much in line with how modern psychology recognizes the importance of our attitude and belief system (schemata).

Beyond religion with all that it offers some people, there is the broad sense of spirituality or faith that is an outgrowth of one's beliefs about life. This can have an impact not only on how we process potentially stressful events but also on how we interact with patients. For our purposes here, I mean "faith" in the broadest sense of the term.

The Sanskrit word for "faith" is *visvas*, which literally translated means "to have trust, to breathe freely, to be without fear." Being able to offer yourself, your colleagues, and your patients encounters marked by such "psychological space" can make all the difference. It is irrelevant whether we say that the approach is based on our faith, attitude, outlook, or the more inclusive term "inner life."

The "inner life" or "interior life" is what spiritual figures point to as a place where ego strength, simplicity, freedom, and truth flourish. It is the setting in which deeply felt needs are experienced and addressed; these include the following:

A need for permanence in a civilization of transience;

A need for the Absolute when all else is becoming relative;

A need for silence in the midst of noise;

A need for gratuitousness in the face of unbelievable greed;

A need for poverty amid the flaunting of wealth;

A need for contemplation in a century of action, for without contemplation, action risks becoming mere agitation;

A need for communication in a universe content with entertainment and sensationalism;

A need for peace amid today's universal outbursts of violence;

A need for quality to counterbalance the increasingly prevalent response to quantity;

A need for humility to counteract the arrogance of power and science;

A need for human warmth when everything is being rationalized or computerized;

A need to belong to a small group rather than to be part of the crowd;

A need for slowness to compensate the present eagerness for
speed;

A need for truth when the real meaning of words is distorted in
political speeches and sometimes even in religious discourses;

A need for transparency when everything seems opaque.

Yes, a need for *the interior life. . . .*[9]

"The interior life" includes those psychological and spiritual factors
that provide us with inner strength, a sound attitude, and a sense of honesty or transparency. Different traditions encourage various approaches
to strengthen or deepen the inner life.

> Our "interior," "inner," or "spiritual" life must take into account
> the needs and tendencies of the whole person. In addition,
> each of us as individuals is unique and therefore must respond
> in accord with his or her own uniqueness. Yet, even though
> this be the case, in the broad sense, there are several attitudes/
> behaviors as well as individual and communal actions that are
> capable of nurturing the "spiritual" dimension of life.[10]

Included among them, the ones that do have great psychological value
and are therefore of interest to us here—whether we are persons of a
specific faith or not—are *silence and solitude, friendship and community*, and
listening and reflection.

Although this list could be made much longer, these three essential
elements of the core spiritual practices have especially sound psychological value for persons seeking to be centered in life in a way that helps
them meet and learn from the necessary stresses in life and to avoid the
unnecessary ones. However, the basis of all of them is a recognition that,
as Abraham Joshua Heschel notes, the inner life "requires education,
training, reflection, contemplation. It is not enough to join others; it is
necessary to build a sanctuary within, brick by brick."[11] Otherwise, we
will be drawn to settle for so little in life and call this "practicality." For
instance, in a similar vein, Heschel also cautions, "People are anxious to
save up financial means for old age; they should also be anxious to prepare a spiritual means for old age. . . . Wisdom, maturity, tranquility do
not come all of a sudden when we retire. . . ."[12]

This latter quote by Heschel came back to me a number of years
ago during one of my regular visits to a mentor. The sessions I had
with him helped me keep perspective. At the time (as now), I was in

the process of helping other health professionals face their own challenges, darkness, stress, and changes. As one might expect, helping them face their own stress, anxiety, despair, and darkness was also dangerous for me. My mentor knew this and called me not to retreat but to go deeper in my own life. The interaction between the two of us can be described as follows:

> Several months ago I was walking with a … mentor through the Virginia countryside on a sunny crisp winter day. About half-way through our usual route along the Shenandoah River, he surprised me with the comment: "I think now may be a good time for you to take your [inner] life more seriously."
>
> Although the statement seemed quite accurate to me at the time, later I wondered why I had not reacted more defensively to it. After all, for almost two years I had been driving one and one-half hours each way, every six weeks or so, to see him. I really felt I had been investing good time and energy in being more open to the deeper elements in my life. So, my natural response could well have been: "Well, what do you think I have been doing?"
>
> However, I think the ideal timing and accuracy of his comment, as well as the trust I had in him and our relationship, made me see his words much differently. What I instantly felt he was trying to tell me was that it was time to leap more freely and deeply into what was truly important in life.[13]

By this I think he meant that I needed to be involved in a three-fold movement to be clearer as to (1) what was the meaning that drove my work as a caregiver for other caregivers and what also provided a theme and purpose for my personal life; (2) how I could continue to care for others in a professional yet deeply compassionate manner; and (3) how I could truly nurture my own interior life through creative, new, disciplined, and simple ways.

Upon reflection, I recognized that to accomplish this I would need to be more aware of the very things to which I had encouraged others to be sensitive in strengthening their inner lives. These steps to a deeper and more resilient self would require an awareness on my part of the aforementioned key aspects of the inner, interior, or spiritual life. And, the first one, *silence and solitude*, would be especially important.

Silence and Solitude

The value of silence and solitude has recently been better recognized for its purely psychological worth due to the work of psychiatrist Anthony Storr. In his work *On Solitude*, he notes the following:

> Modern psychotherapists, including myself have taken as their criterion of emotional maturity the capacity of the individual to make mature relationships on equal terms. With few exceptions, psychotherapists have omitted to consider the fact that the capacity to be alone is also an aspect of emotional maturity.[14]

In this volume, he presents Admiral Byrd as an example of someone who searched for solitude. Byrd appreciated its value, as well as the silence he experienced as part and parcel of the experience. Reflecting on his solo Antarctic expedition in the winter of 1934, Byrd wrote the following:

> Aside from the meteorological and auroral work, I had no important purposes. . . . Nothing whatsoever, except one man's desire to know that kind of experience to the full, to be by himself for a while and to taste peace and quiet and solitude long enough to find out how good they really are. . . . I wanted something more than just privacy in the geographical sense. I wanted to sink roots into some replenishing philosophy. . . . I did take away something that I had not fully possessed before: appreciation of the sheer beauty and miracle of being alive, and a humble set of values. . . . Civilization has not altered my ideas. I live more simply now, and with more peace.[15]

From a spiritual standpoint, long before Storr and other psychiatrists and psychologists wrote positively about silence and solitude, all the major religions pointed out the value of taking out time to retreat from activity. This is clearly reflected in the writings of contemporary spiritual figures. For instance, Henri Nouwen, a Catholic spiritual writer (and incidentally also a psychologist), notes in his book *Way of the Heart* that silence and solitude are the furnace in which transformation takes place.[16]

In his book *The Tibetan Book of Living and Dying*, contemporary Buddhist author Sogyal Rinpoche frames such periods of silence as "meditation." He points out that slowing down the pace of our lives by ensuring we have time to stop, breathe, slow down, and see how habits and compulsions have quietly strangled us is essential. He writes the following:

> We are already perfectly trained . . . trained to get jealous, trained to grasp, trained to be anxious and sad and desperate and greedy, trained to react angrily to whatever provokes us. We are trained . . . to such an extent that these negative emotions rise spontaneously, without our even trying to generate them. . . . However if we devote the mind in meditation to the task of freeing itself from illusions, we will find that with time, patience, discipline, and the right training, our mind will begin to unknot itself and know the essential bliss and clarity.[17]

He then goes on to say the following:

> The gift of learning to meditate is the greatest gift you can give yourself in this life. For it is only through meditation that you can understand the journey to discover your true nature, and so find the stability and confidence you will need to live, and die, well. Meditation is the road to enlightenment. . . .
>
> Our lives are lived in intense and anxious struggle, in a swirl of speed and aggression, in competing, grasping, possessing, and achieving, forever burdening ourselves with extraneous activities and preoccupations. Meditation is the exact opposite.[18]

Orthodox Rabbi Aryeh Kaplan expresses a similar positive sentiment regarding meditation in his book *Meditation and Kabbalah*. In it, he ties meditation to a number of sources, indicating the late eighteenth century-early nineteenth century as its most popular period. He also acknowledges the fact that technique is similar throughout different world religions and points out that in Judaism there is a lack of awareness of this tradition of meditation for all practicing Jews:

> With the spread of the Hasidic movement in the Eighteenth Century, a number of meditative techniques became more popular, especially those centered around the formal prayer service. This reached its zenith in the teachings of Rabbi Nachman of Breslov (1772–1810), who discusses

meditation in considerable length. He developed a system that could be used by the masses, and it was primarily for this reason that Rabbi Nachman's teachings met with much harsh opposition.

One of the problems in discussing meditation, either in Hebrew or in English, is the fact that there exists only a very limited vocabulary with which to express the various "technical" terms. . . .

Many people [also] express surprise that the Jewish tradition contains a formal meditative system, that, at least in its outward manifestations, does resemble some of the Eastern systems. This resemblance was first noted in Zohar, which recognized the merit of the Eastern systems, but warned against their use.

The fact that different systems resemble each other is only a reflection on the veracity of the technique, which is primarily one of spiritual liberation. The fact that other religions make use of it is of no more consequence than the fact that they also engage in prayer and worship. This does not make Jewish worship and prayer any less meaningful or unique, and the same is true of meditation. It is basically a technique for releasing oneself from the bonds of one's physical nature. Where one goes from there depends upon the system used.[19]

Whether we are Buddhist, Muslim, Jewish, Christian, Hindu, or religious at all, though, the point made when we speak about time in silence and solitude or formal meditation is that there is a benefit—especially for those working in the intense health care setting today. For instance, Clark Strand, a former Zen Buddhist monk, wrote *The Wooden Bowl*, which is about taking out time for meditation even though you are no longer holding onto a religious or philosophical ideology:

All I wanted in the first place was to find the simple truth about who we are and how we ought to live. . . . I asked myself one question: Was there a way for people to slow down and experience themselves, their lives, and other people in the present moment. . . . The only thing [meditation] requires is that you be willing to remain a beginner, that you forgo achieving any expert status. . . . In other words, it requires you to maintain a spirit of lightness and friendliness with regard to what you are doing. It's nothing special, but it works.[20]

In extolling the value of being a meditative person—whether you are religious or not does not matter in his mind—Strand goes on to say what he believes it offers all of us:

Perhaps you have had the experience of waking well-rested on a Saturday morning. Your mind is alert but you have not yet begun to think about the day. The sun is shining in the yard and all around you is perfectly clear morning light. That alertness sustains itself without even trying. You may not even notice it except for the feeling of being rested and ready for the day.

The experience of meditation is something like that. When you meditate you are not trying to have any particular experience. You are simply awake. After having counted your breath from one to four for several minutes, quite without having aimed at that experience, you start to feel a kind of clarity and space surrounding each number as you count. It feels a little like having enough space to think, enough room to move and breathe, or simply "be."[21]

Still, the questions remain as to how we do it, what is the cost involved in terms of time, and loss of illusions about ourselves and the benefits that are possible so we can see the effort as being worthwhile. As I have noted elsewhere:

We must be able to hear our own inner voice instead of only our anxieties and the myriad fearful and negative voices that fill our outer world at home, in the classroom, at places of amusement, [in the hospital], and that even dominate our places of worship! But in today's active life, where and when do we find such space? Furthermore, given our lack of experience with it, how will we spend this time alone in a way that is renewing? We don't want to let it be just a time for moody introspection or vengeful musings about how we have been mistreated in life. . . .

The benefits are certainly there if we approach such a place, not with a sense of duty, but as a time for returning to our self; it will become a gentle place of reassurance, reassessment and peace. Time spent in silence and solitude on a regular basis can affect us in the following ways:

Sharpen our sense of clarity about the life we are living and the choices we are making

Enhance our attitude of simplicity

Increase our humility and help us avoid unnecessary arrogance by allowing time to examine the defenses and games we play (these often surface for us to see during quiet times)

Let us enjoy our relationship with ourselves more

Decrease our dependence on the reinforcement of others

Enable us to recognize our own areas of anger, entitlement, greed, cowardice (given the opportunity to quietly review the day's activities and our reaction to them)

Protect our own inner fire so that we can reach out without being pulled down

Help us accept change and loss

Make us more sensitive to the compulsions in our lives

Experience the importance of love and acceptance (which are fruits of the contemplative life) and acknowledge the silliness and waste involved in condemning self and judging others

Allow us to hear the gentle inner voice that reflects the spiritual sound of authenticity . . . and

Help us to respect the need to take time to strengthen our own inner space so that we can, in turn, be more sensitive to the . . . presence of others. . . .

In other words, taking quiet time in solitude and silence during each day can provide us with a place to breathe deeply. . . . Yet, even when we know the true value of silence and solitude, we run from it. For us, to value the quiet in our lives, we must know not only what these periods can do for us but also . . . be able to really appreciate *what price they may extract from us*. Otherwise, we will just continue to speak about silence and solitude wistfully as something wonderful and never enjoy what this well of truth and support can offer us.[22]

Recognizing the Challenges of Silence and Solitude

People always make time for what they want to do. When the schedule
is full, they may get up early, stay up late, or set aside periods during the
day—even if it turns out to limit their lunch break. So, why would we
not want to set aside time for quiet periods if we feel they really have
so many benefits?

Resistance to Solitude

Silence speaks eloquently in solitude; listening quietly to our
hearts allows us to walk unprotected and unguarded with the
Truth in our inner "garden." However, this time of quiet listening may also present us with a challenge: It may bring us to
a place of loneliness and vulnerability, open us to a new recognition of hidden lies. So, although the process of taking time
away from our daily activities is essential and good, there are
elements with which we will find it difficult to deal once we
embrace silence and solitude. We should know about this challenging reality so that the unconscious hesitancy to take quiet
time doesn't surprise us and totally undermine our efforts to
seek solitude. Time away for reflection is too valuable to lose
because of ignorance or hidden anxiety.

Our natural tendency is to actively avoid silence and time
alone. Distracting and amusing ourselves with activities is a
much more common practice than being involved on a regular
basis in the process of reflection. . . . [It] confronts us with the
awkward way we often live out our days; likewise, in silence,
we are reminded of our mortality. Consequently, talking about
[meditation] is a lot easier than [meditating]. Thus, when we
seek to establish a life of reflection or further develop the . . .
life [of silence and solitude] we have, we must realize that the
process won't go as smoothly as we'd like. A road sign at the
beginning of a highway construction site outside of Washington, D.C. warns:

BE PREPARED TO BE FRUSTRATED!

As we travel along the roadway of [meditation], the same advice
is often appropriate. The difficult experiences we encounter
during periods of solitude need not be considered negative
even if initially we feel that they are. If we neither avoid nor

run away from them, we can learn to understand and appreciate the constructive moments of our periods of loneliness, vulnerability and discovery.

For instance, a number of years ago, as I was walking down a winding Virginia road with a mentor, I shared with him an unusual experience I had during my quiet time. I said to him, "My life is basically quite good. I don't feel deprived or needy. Instead, most of the time I feel grateful and challenged. However, lately in my quiet time of reflection, I have felt a sense of wistful loneliness, like something was missing. I felt a light ache of emptiness passing through my stomach . . . that something real, important and basic was missing, and I deeply yearned for it—whatever this 'it' was."

His response surprised me. He did not brush off my experience as of no consequence, advise that it would pass shortly or tell me how to combat it. Instead he said, "That's good. The loneliness that you describe is meant to remind you that your heart will not be ultimately satisfied by anyone or anything now in this life. Your loneliness also reminds you that even though you may distract yourself with many things and people—even lovely ones—your sense of being at home can only be given by something deeper, greater.

"And so, the loneliness will allow you to enjoy people, things and life in general *in their proper perspective*. As a result, you can enjoy the people and gifts in life, but they will not become idols for you because your loneliness will teach you. . . .

"Then, rather than being tempted to 'set up tents' prematurely when you have wonderful experiences or relationships, you will have the freedom to enjoy them without being captured and controlled by your desire for them. Therefore, the loneliness will keep your heart open, aware; your journey will continue with a sense of passion and expectancy. That is, if you let it and don't try to avoid or 'medicate' such initially troubling feelings with activities, distractions or work."

Andrew Harvey, in his famous book *A Journey in Ladakh*, approaches this feeling from a Buddhist perspective by offering a response he received from someone with whom he shared a similar situation:

As we parted, he hugged me and said, "You smile a great deal and you listen well, but I see that somewhere you are sad. I see that nothing has satisfied you. . . ."

I started to protest.

"No," he said, "nothing has satisfied you, not your work, not your friendships, not all your learning and travelling. And that is good. You are ready to learn something new. Your sadness has made you empty; your sadness has made you open!"[23]

A Psychological Vacuum

As well as opening us to loneliness and vulnerability, silence and solitude can form a psychological vacuum into which many feelings, memories, and awarenesses (which lie just below the surface in the preconscious) may be encouraged to surface. At such times as these, we are being called in reflection . . . to face the truths about ourselves that for some unconscious reason we may have put aside, denied, or diminished.

Having such truths surface is not terrible, of course, especially if we remember that many of these insights will actually be helpful rather than harmful. The only "damage" is that which will be suffered by the false image of ourselves that we have created because we have not been willing to trust in our own inherent value. So by spending time in silence and solitude, we will be able to see the extent to which our self-worth has, to this point, been built upon a foundation of sand. We will come to recognize that our sense of self-worth is dependent in an exaggerated way on praise by others, positive experiences we have (including ones in prayer and meditation), and a list of other past achievements. Though unpleasant, finding out this truth is still quite life-giving. Such an epiphany allows us to rediscover a sense of self and worth grounded in true self-respect. We then can come to understand that real self-respect is based on a deep, concrete trust in the inherent spiritual value of being a human person rather than on specific accomplishments or the reception of kudos from others.

Arriving at this point of insight is not a magical process. The desire to be a person who is solidly aware of self-worth no matter what others say or do, no matter what mistakes or shameful things we might do, cannot thrive just as a wishful thought. It has to be welcomed and passionately sought in silence and solitude, that place in which a strong and healthy attitude toward *all* of life is formed.[24]

Once we consider taking out the time to sit in silence and solitude or *zazen* in a group, we may then come up with another set of objections:

The *first objection* is: "When I quiet down and try to enjoy the silence, all I do is hear the noise of my thoughts and worries. So I know I'm not made for meditation or reflection." This is a typical objection of beginners. It needs to be handled, otherwise we will quit after a couple of minutes, no matter how many times we try.

The reality is that most of us hear noise in our minds all day long. When we sit in silence, the first important bit of information we get is to learn how preoccupied we are with so many things. Knowing this is helpful because it

- Helps us let the static expend itself. (Given a chance, after a while our mind clams down.)
- Gives us some indication of the type of worries we have about which we feel helpless or anxious. (We get a chance to hear what we are continually thinking.)
- Prepares us to empty our minds so we can breathe deeply, relax, and experience "the now" rather than always being caught in the past or preoccupied with the future.

So, expecting the noise and letting it move through us are two ways we can meet the objection that we are not suited or able to quietly reflect or meditate. The reality we must remember is: Many people with our personality type have found meditation wonderfully helpful. It is not just a certain type of person.

A *second objection* is: "Meditation or reflection is too hard and alien. I'm not a yogi and have found meditation or even quiet prayer uncomfortable." The response to this is simple:

- Find a quiet place (alone if possible).
- Sit up straight.
- Close your eyes or keep them slightly open looking a few feet in front of you.

- Count slow, naturally exhaled breaths from one to four and repeat the process.
- Relax and let stray thoughts move through you like a slow-moving train, repeating themes; observe objectively then let them go. . . .
- Experience living in the now.

A *third objection* comes in the form of a question: "What will this time do for me? I'm a busy person and time is too precious for me to deal with impractical exercises." There are many responses to this. For our purposes here—namely, the desire to change, grow, and be more free—the following are especially relevant:

- When we are quiet we are able to experience all of the pulls, anxieties, and conditioned responses we have going on all day but may fail to notice. So, at the very lest it informs us of the nature of the blocks we have to feeling at ease, flexible, open, and ready to change when necessary.
- Not only will we be able to see what absorbs us but how things we didn't realize have become our most important reference point or center of psychological/spiritual gravity.
- Once we have this information we can take note of it and reflect on it mentally, in journaling, or with a mentor during other periods outside of the quiet time.
- Also, the peaceful times when we sit and reflect physically stop us from running, running, running, without taking a breath, and so experience what it means to be alive and, in the process, ask ourselves if that is where we want to focus our lives.

If it sounds like I am putting great emphasis on quiet time, I am. I have found if we give some space to ourselves and try not to judge ourselves and others harshly, and avoid panicking or trying to immediately solve a problem, but instead calm ourselves down, we will learn not to jump to quick conclusions; our usual ways of doing business (our programming) will not take hold. This will allow our habits to loosen their hold on us so we can see life—including ourselves—differently.

When people do express their gratitude for my recommendation that they take at least two minutes a day for quiet

reflection first thing in the morning, they often report extending it to twenty minutes. Then they try to find another ten
minutes during the day to reconnect with the experience and
find another few minutes in the evening to become tranquil,
give closure, and release the day before they go to sleep.

In guiding others toward using meditation as a building
block to enable change, one of the other things I also notice is
that it loosens people up throughout their whole day—not just
during the reflection period. The more we allow our thoughts
to inform, rather than frighten, depress, or anger us, the less we
are grasped by our [rigid] thinking and interpretations. We are
not in a vise but are instead free to use our power of observation, analysis, and curiosity to help us learn valuable lessons
about life. Meditation not only frees us to be open during the
period of reflection, it also produces an attitude that makes us
less defensive and more intrigued with stumbles as well as tri-
umphs. It can positively contaminate our day![25]

Friendship and Community

As well as silence and solitude, one of the other key aspects of the inner
life is to have a well-rounded circle of friends. Anthropologist Margaret Meade once noted that "One of the oldest human needs is having someone to wonder where you are when you don't come home
at night."[26] Psychology has long emphasized the need to relate as a
key element of health and happiness. For all major spiritual traditions,
"community" is an essential element. Yet, who is in that community is
just as significant as the recognition that we should be part of one. As
psychologist and spiritual writer Henri Nouwen recognizes: "We can
take a lot of physical and even mental pain when we know that it truly
makes us a part of the life we live together in the world. But when we
feel cut off from the human family, we quickly lose heart."[27] An absence
of at least one significant friend may also have physical consequences.

Redford Williams, M.D., of Duke University, tracked almost
1,400 men and women who underwent coronary angiograms
and were found to have at least one severely blocked coronary
artery. After five years, those who were unmarried and who

did not have at least one close confidante were over three times more likely to have died than people who were married, had one or more confidantes, or both.[28]

In my work,[29] I have found that for the circle to be rich, we need, at the very least, four "types" or "voices" (because one friend may play different beneficial roles at different points in our lives) among them. They are the prophet, the cheerleader, the harasser, and the guide. By having these "voices" in our lives, the chances are greater that we will be able to maintain a sense of perspective, openness, and balance. A brief description of each follows[30]:

The Prophet
The first of these voices which help us maintain balance and have a sense of openness is the one I shall refer to as the prophet. Contrary to what one might imagine, prophetic friends need not look or behave any differently than other types of persons who are close to us. . . . The true prophet's voice is often quiet and fleeting, but nonetheless strong. She or he is living an honest courageous life guided by truth and compassion. . . . They are trying to live out the truth, and whether knowingly or not, they follow the advice of Gandhi: "Let our first act every morning be this resolve: I shall not fear anyone on earth. I shall fear only God. I shall not bear ill-will toward anyone. I shall conquer untruth by truth and in resisting untruth, I shall put up with all suffering."

The message of prophets often involves discomfort or pain, not masochistic pain but real pain. Often they do not directly produce conflict. Instead, like leaders in the non-violent movement, they "merely" set the stage for it, as is pointed out in the following words of Martin Luther King, Jr.:

We who engage in nonviolent, direct action are
Not the creators of tension. We merely bring to
The surface the hidden tension that is already
alive. We bring it out in the open, where it can be
seen and dealt with. Like a boil that can never be
cured so long as it is covered up but must be
opened with all its ugliness to the natural
medicines of air and light, injustice must be exposed, with all the tension its exposure creates,

to the light of human conscience and the air of
national opinion before it can be cured.

Having someone prophetic in our lives is never easy. No matter how positive we may believe the ultimate consequences
will be for us, many of us still shy away from prophetic mes-
sages and would readily agree with Henry Thoreau: "If you see
someone coming to do you a good deed, run for your life!"
However, to seek comfort in lieu of the truth may mean that
in an effort to avoid pain, we will also avoid responding to
opportunities of real value, real life. We will merely exist and
eventually die without having ever really lived. . . . Prophets
point! They point to the fact that it doesn't matter whether
pleasure or pain is involved, the only thing that matters is . . .
that we seek to see and live "the truth" because only it will
set us free.

In doing this, prophets challenge us to look at how we are
living our lives, to ask ourselves: "To what voices am I listening
when I form my attitudes and take my actions each day?"

The Cheerleader

Ironically, one of the most controversial suggestions I might
make with respect to friendship is to suggest we all need
"cheerleaders." . . . Some might say that to encourage this type
of friend is to run the risk of narcissism and denial. However,
to balance the prophetic voices . . . we also need unabashed,
enthusiastic, unconditional acceptance by certain people in
our lives. Prophecy can and should instill appropriate guilt to
break through the crusts of our denial. But guilt cannot sustain
us for long. While guilt will push us to do good things because
they are right, love encourages us to do the right thing because
it is natural.

We can't go it alone. We need a balance of support. We
need encouragement and acceptance as much as we need the
criticism and feedback that are difficult to hear. Burnout is
always around the corner when we don't have people who are
ready to encourage us, see our gifts clearly, and be there for us
when our involvement with people, their sometimes unrealistic demands, and our own crazy expectations for ourselves,
threaten to pull us down. . . . So, while having buoyantly sup-

portive friends may seem like a luxury, make no mistake about it—it is a necessity that is not to be taken lightly. The "interpersonal roads" of time are strewn with well-meaning helpers who tried to survive without such support. Encouragement is a gift that should be treasured in today's stressful, anxious, complex world because the seeds of involvement and the seeds of burnout are the same. To be involved is to risk. And to risk without the presence of solidly supportive friends is foolhardy and dangerous.

The Harasser

When singer-activist Joan Baez was asked her opinion about Thomas Merton, one of the things she said was that he was different than many of the phony gurus she had encountered in her travels. She said that although Merton took important things seriously in his life, he didn't take himself too seriously. She indicated that he knew how to laugh at situations and particularly at himself. . . .[31] "Harassers" help us to laugh at ourselves and to avoid the emotional burnout resulting from having the unrealistic expectation that people will always follow our guidance or appreciate what we do for them. This type of friend helps us regain and maintain perspective (so we don't unnecessarily waste valuable energy). This is truly a gift for which we can be thankful.

Spiritual Guides

The three types of friends we've looked at thus far are each part of a necessary community. The prophet enhances our sense of single-heartedness. The cheerleader generously showers us with the support we feel we need. The harasser encourages us to maintain a sense of proper perspective. Complementing these three is a cluster that, for lack of a better name, shall be referred to as "spiritual guides" . . . guides listen to us carefully and don't accept the "manifest content" (what we say and do) as being equal to the "total content" (our actual intentions plus our statements and actions). Instead, they search and look for nuances in what we share with them to help us to uncover some of the "voices" that are unconsciously guiding our lives, especially the ones that undermine our trust in God and make us hesitant, anxious, fearful, and willful.

To determine whether or how these voices are in our lives, several questions or statements about the composition of our circle of friends might be helpful:

- Do I have people with whom I can simply be myself?
- What type of friends do I value most? Why?
- What do I feel are the main qualities of friendship?
- List and briefly describe the friends who are now in my life.
- Describe ones who are no longer alive or present to me now but who have made an impact on my life. Why do I think they made such a difference in my life?
- Among my circle of friends, who are my personal heroes or role models?
- Who are the prophets in my life? In other words, who confronts me with the question: To what voices am I responding in life?
- Who helps me see my relationships, mission in life, and self-image more clearly? How do they accomplish this?
- Who encourages me in a genuine way through praise and a nurturing spirit?
- Who teases me into gaining a new perspective when I am too preoccupied or tied up in myself? . . .
- When and with whom do I play different (prophetic, supportive . . .) roles as a friend? How do people receive such interactions?[32]

Psychologically and spiritually, having a healthy and balanced circle of friends can aid in stress prevention and personal/professional growth. This is an obvious reality. The important point here is that with some attention to this area, we can immeasurably improve the role that encouraging, challenging, and guiding friendships can have in our lives.

Listening and Reflection

Listening to the people around us and opening ourselves to what we hear coming from within us may cause us some shame and emotional pain at first if we are really honest. However, just as we should not turn our back on others who would help us see the truth, we must also have the patience and fortitude to "just sit" and be quiet when all that comes from within rises to the surface. As Achaan Chah advises:

> Just go into the room and put one chair in the center. Take the one seat in the center of the room, open the doors and windows, and see who comes to visit. You will witness all kinds of scenes and actors, all kinds of temptations and stories, everything imaginable. Your only job is to stay in your seat. You will see it all arise and pass, and out of this wisdom and understanding will come.[33]

By having a listening spirit, we recognize that we must face things directly. The American Buddhist nun Pema Chodron addresses this issue in her book *When Things Fall Apart*. She writes: "The trick is to keep exploring and not bail out, even when we find out something is not what we thought . . . [a] sign of health is that we don't become undone by fear and trembling, but we take it as a message that it's time to stop struggling and look directly at what's threatening us."[34]

Being as open as we can in both meditation and in our relationships can teach us a great deal about ourselves if we really "listen" "(a very important word) to the people and the world around us" and by opening ourselves "despite the pain that may be associated with it to the possibilities . . . that fill and surround us and sometimes . . . even come kicking, scratching, or begging at our door."[35] And so, what we are speaking about here in the effort to be a true listener to whatever provides greater awareness and inner strength is not something to be taken lightly. This can be put another way:

> The interior life then is not an imaginary or psychotic world. It is not a place to run to so we can pout, brood, fantasize revenge, or to ruminate over things as a way to mentally beat ourselves up. Instead, as we have seen, it is a place of self-knowledge, self-nurturance, challenge, and solid peace. It is a place that will not only be our strength but also one that we can offer to others. When our interior life is strong, our attitude toward others is gentle. When our inner life feels nourished, our hearts can be open to others' pain.

In a reflection on our time together, one person whom I journeyed with said: "And what will I leave behind from our relationship: my 'stuckness,' my unconsciousness, my shame and guilt, my repressed pain, resentment and depression....And what will I take with me? What will be awakened through the gift of our relationship? My playfulness, my love of life, my sense of wonder, my gratitude, my openness, and my wholeness."

Unfortunately, though, our inner life is often infected by some of the negative "atmosphere" of our upbringing. For instance, Gorky in his autobiography said: "Grandfather's house was filled with a choking fog of mutual hostility. It poisoned the grown-ups and even infected the children."[36]

Our response to such influences is to build a persona inside that is filled with fear, hesitancy, prickliness, and anger—not a very gentle place for us to center ourselves.

Moreover, when our inner life is narrow and distorted, our understanding, appreciation, and grasp of life also suffer dramatically. Carl Jung, the famous Swiss psychiatrist, put it in these terms:

> People become neurotic when they content
> themselves with inadequate or wrong answers
> to the question of life. They seek position, mar-
> riage, reputation, outward success or money,
> and remain unhappy and neurotic even when
> they have attained what they were seeking.
> Such people are usually confined within too
> narrow a spiritual horizon.... If they are enabled
> to develop more spacious personalities, the
> neurosis generally disappears.

What he is speaking about here is the inner life, the spiritual life, the one we all long for as a way of finding a deep well within ourselves which will remain calm and pure no matter how stormy, violent, or polluted the interpersonal "weather" around us becomes.

The inner life is important because it impacts every aspect of our living since we interpret all aspects of life via this inner sense of self and the world. For instance, one person who was once sexually abused at a very young age said at the end of therapy that, early in her life, transitions seemed abrupt, fearful, and everything seemed worse after them. "Now that I am in a different place in my heart," she said, "transitions are to be reached out to with wonder and awe."

The state of our interior life *does* make a difference to others. When we have a gentle, healthy, and strong inner life, we are part of the healing stillness in the world which offers places of hope to all who suffer and yearn for justice, solace, and encouragement. But if we, like so many others, do not feel at home within ourselves, and by ourselves, we will then add to the sense in the world that nowhere is there a safe and good place.

This is a very dangerous situation not only for us but also for the young who follow and try to model themselves after us. Ten years ago one pediatrician noted to me that she saw the light go out in the eyes of many fifth and sixth graders—now she sees this same sad shroud over their spontaneity in the second and third grades.

So, we need to build our inner life. . . .[37]

However, being a listening-reflective person does take some sense of structured intention rather than just motivation and good will. It involves

1. Finding time to reflect
2. Selecting meaningful events in our day and life to reflect upon
3. Entering those events by reliving them in our minds
4. Given our desires, goals, and philosophy of life, to learn what we can from these events
5. Enlivening the learning through action

An elaboration of the five-step process follows:

Time: A little time is needed to reflect on one's day. If we rush through life, without thought we will know it. One sign we are doing this is the statement: "Where did the time go?" When our life is passing like a blur, it does not mean that we live very *active* lives. What it does show is that we are leading *busy* lives. The difference between "active" and "busy" is that the former includes reflection and is directed, whereas the busy life feels out of control and does not seem purposeful or meaningful.

Select: To make our reflection useful and not just a time to preoccupy ourselves, to worry, or to let our mind wander, we should pick

out *specific* events or interactions during the day that caused a significant reaction.

Enter: Then we should put ourselves back into the events so we
can relive them. This time as we experience it we can observe our reactions, note them, and see what themes or understanding we can glean.
(Remember, do not *blame* others or *condemn* self, just neutrally observe
and seek to analyze.)

Learn: Given what we understand and what our core beliefs (psychological or spiritual) are about life, what did we learn from this reflection? Often when we have values, we can see how we followed those
values or ignored them.

Action: Finally, learning is only important when it changes the way
we live. How we will act on our new learning is essential. And it cannot be action that is immature such as, when you feel a person has let
you down, making the vow, *I'll never trust him again!* Instead, using the
example just cited, you must see what about the interaction led you to
be naïve and to put more trust in a certain person than he or she could
bear. So, in other words, action must be based on insight that we have
about our *own* behavior, beliefs, and thoughts. Otherwise, the results
will be just a sophisticated form of pouting, projecting, and avoidance
of self-understanding.[38]

When we become true listeners, we practice being people who
recognize that there are many voices calling to us of which we are not
aware. The sources of them may be good in their own way and include
the desire to succeed, be well off financially, be admired, be spectacu-
larly effective, or be loved. The sources can be career, family upbringing, society, the health care system, politics, or culture. The important
thing when we make daily decisions and decisions that affect us in the
long run is to know which ones are primary at any given time so we
can more clearly decide, based on this knowledge, what we wish to do
in any given situation. And so, one of the positive outcomes of a strong
inner life is such a level of self-awareness.

Naturally, there are many other elements and "fruits" of a strong
inner life. As has been noted, having a strong community of friends
and knowing the benefit of taking out time in silence and solitude
certainly are among them. Taking out time to further explore your history and current sense of the role of religion and/or spirituality in your
life, regardless of whether you are presently a person of faith, can be
helpful.[39] To assist in this, a guide to clarifying your spiritual life map is

Table 3-1 Clarifying Your Spiritual Life Map

---

1. Do you consider yourself a spiritual person? If so, explain.
2. What role did spirituality and/or religion play in your family growing up? What role does it play now?
3. When the word "God" is used, what images come to mind?
4. When you are under stress, depressed, anxious, lost, angry, joyful, happy, elated, or experiencing other strong emotions, does God or spirituality play a role for you when these states are present?
5. If you are part of an organized religion, how does this affect the way you function as a physician, nurse, or allied health professional? How does it affect your personal life?
6. If you have a personal relationship with God, how does this affect the way you live your life?
7. What type of spiritual practices do you have, and has their meaningfulness and/or form changed in recent years?
8. Do you seek to read the sacred scripture of one or more of the major world religions or spiritual books? What do you seek to get out of them? How has this reading list changed over the years?
9. Given your own beliefs, how do you interact with others of different beliefs? Do you find their literature, practices, or beliefs a help to you in any way?
10. When you are under stress, what parts of your spirituality—if any—provide you with a sense of relief and perspective?

---

provided here to offer ideas (Table 3-1). No matter how you begin to sensitize yourself to this area, the information can provide additional self-knowledge and set the stage for the development of a richer self-care protocol.

Objectives of Chapter Three

- Appreciate the potential roles of both religion and spirituality in the life of the physician, nurse, and allied health professional
- Understand the possible needs that encourage people to seek an "interior life"
- Appreciate both the value and some of the major resistances to meditation
- Learn one basic approach to meditation
- Be familiar with four different "voices" that should be in our circle of friends so that we are able to better maintain perspec-

tive and be both encouraged and challenged in our personal
and professional lives
- Know how to question ourselves to determine if the composition of our circle of friends is as complete as is needed
- Be aware of one structural listening-reflective approach and
the five elements it involves if it is to have practical impact in
our professional and personal lives
- Know how to begin an assessment of your own spiritual/reli-
gious life map

Additional Books to Consider

There are different approaches to spiritual reading, including reading inner journeys (journals or autobiographical fragments), biog-
raphies/autobiographies, quotes from spiritual masters, wisdom from
the East, Western Spirituality, and spiritual/self-help/new age material.
The composition or approach depends on whether you are religious,
the faith group to which you belong, whether you are a "searcher"
and have no religious affiliation, and how interested you are in using
a broad or focused approach. Some samples of the types of books just
mentioned include inner journeys—Kathleen Norris' *Dakota*, Mitch
Albom's *Tuesdays with Morrie*, Annie Dillard's *The Writing Life*, Anne
LaMott's *Traveling Mercies*, and Andrew Harvey's *A Journey in Ladakh*;
contemporary biographies/autobiographies—Michael Mott's *The Seven
Mountains of Thomas Merton*, David Chadwick's *A Crooked Cucumber: The
Life and Zen Teachings of Shunryu Suzuki*, and the Dalai Lama's *Freedom
in Exile*; quotes from the spiritual sages—Anthony deMello's *One Min-
ute Wisdom* and Abraham Heschel's *I Asked for Wonder*; wisdom from the
East—Pema Chodron's *When Things Fall Apart*, Jack Kornfield's *A Path
with Heart*, and Sogyal Rinpoche's *The Tibetan Book of Living and Dying*,
Western spirituality—Henri Nouwen's *Reaching Out*, Thomas Merton's
New Seeds of Contemplation, Kenneth Leech's *True Prayer*, Mary Elizabeth
O'Brien's *Spirituality for Nurses* (Second Edition), B. Barnum's *Spiritual-
ity for Nurses* (Second Edition), Beverly Eanes, Lee Richmond, and Jean
Link's *What Brings You to Life: Awakening Woman's Spiritual Essence*, and
the Robert J. Wicks books *Riding the Dragon*, *Living a Gentle, Passionate
Life*, *Touching the Holy*, *Everyday Simplicity*, *Living Simply in an Anxious
World*, *Simple Changes*, *Snow Falling on Snow*, and *Seeds of Sensitivity*.

(Note: For a more complete list, you may wish to consult the section "Some Readings I Have Found Helpful" in my book *Riding the Dragon*, pp. 152–157.)

Notes

1. I. Yalom, source unknown.

2. R. Piedmont, "Spiritual Transcendence as a Predictor of Psychosocial Outcome from an Outpatient Substance Abuse Program," *Psychology of Addictive Behaviors* (in press); R. Piedmont, "Spiritual Transcendence and the Scientific Study of Spirituality," *Journal of Rehabilitation*, 67 (2001): 4–14.

3. E. Baker, *Caring for Ourselves* (Washington, DC: American Psychiatric Association, 2003), 95.

4. S. W. Emmett, "Spirituality, Self-Care and the Therapist," *The Perspective: A Professional Journal of the Renfrew Center Foundation*, 5, 10–13.

5. H. Benson, *Timeless Healing: The Power and Biology of Belief*. (New York: Charles Scribner and Sons, 1996).

6. K. Pargament, *The Psychology of Religion and Coping* (New York: Guilford Press, 1997); K. Pargament, "Religious Methods of Coping: Resources for Conservation and Transformation of Significance," in E. P. Shafranske (Ed.), *Religion and the Clinical Practice of Psychology* (Washington, DC: American Psychiatric Association, 1996).

7. R. Hood, B. Spilka, B. Budsberger, and R. Gorsuch, *The Psychology of Religion* (New York: Guilford Press, 1996).

8. The works of Rabbi A. Twerski, M.D., are good follow-up reading on this point.

9. D. Dubois, "Renewal of Prayer," *Lumen Vitae*, 38 (1983): 3: 273–274.

10. R. Wicks, *After 50* (Mahwah, NJ: Paulist Press, 1997), 11–12.

11. A. Heschel, "On Prayer," *Conservative Judaism*, XXV (1970): 1.

12. A. Heschel, *The Insecurity of Freedom* (New York: Farrar, Straus, and Giroux, 1951), 79.

13. R. Wicks, Op. Cit. (1997), 3.

14. A. Storr, *On Solitude* (New York: Bantam, 1988), 18.

15. R. Byrd, *Alone* (New York: G.P. Putnam's Sons, 1938), 7, 9, 62, 63.

16. H. Nouwen, *The Way of the Heart* (New York: Seabury/Harper Collins, 1981), 20.

17. S. Rinpoche, *The Tibetan Book of Living and Dying* (New York: Harper Collins, 2002).

18. Ibid., p. 57.

19. A. Kaplan, *Meditation and Kabbalah* (York Beach, ME: Samuel Weiser, 1982), 3.

20. C. Strand, *The Wooden Bowl* (New York: Hyperion, 1998), 2–3.

21. Ibid., 96.

22. R. Wicks, *Living a Gentle, Passionate Life* (Mahwah, NJ: Paulist Press, 1998), 41–43.

23. A. Harvey, *A Journey in Ladakh* (Boston: Houghton-Mifflin, 1983), 65.

24. R. Wicks, Op. Cit. (1998), 45–49.

25. R. Wicks, *Simple Changes* (Allen, TX: Thomas More, 2000), 52–55.

26. M. Meade, source unknown.

27. H. Nouwen, *Making All Things New* (New York: Harper and Row, 1981), 33.

28. A. Domar, *Self-Nurture* (New York: Penguin Group, 2000), 213.

29. R. Wicks and R. Hamma, *Circle of Friends* (Notre Dame, IN: AMP, 1996); R. Wicks *Touching the Holy: Ordinariness, Self-Esteem, and Friendship* (Notre Dame, IN: AMP, 1992).

30. R. Wicks, Op. Cit. (1992), 96–111.

31. J. Baez in P. Wilkes (Ed.), *Merton: By Those Who Knew Him Best* (Harper: San Francisco, 1984), 45.

32. R. Wicks, Op. Cit. (1997), 69–70.

33. Quoted in J. Kornfield, *A Path with Heart* (New York: Bantam, 1993).

34. P. Chodron, *When Things Fall Apart* (Boston: Shambala, 1997).

35. R. Wicks, Op. Cit. (1997), 14.

36. M. Gorky, *Gorky: My Childhood* (London: Penguin, 1996), 173.

37. R. Wicks, Op. Cit. (1997), 14–16.

38. R. Wicks, Op. Cit. (2000), 57–58.

39. There are sections in the following two books that may be helpful in this regard: J. Ciarrocchi, *Counseling Problem Gamblers: A Self-Regulation Manual for Individuals and Family Therapy* (San Diego, CA: Academic Press, 2002), and R. Wicks, *Seeds of Sensitivity: Deepening Your Spiritual Life* (Notre Dame, IN: AMP, 1995).

FOUR

The Simple Care of a Hopeful Heart

Developing a Personally Designed Self-Care Protocol

**MEDICAL LIBRARY
WESTERN INFIRMARY
GLASGOW**

Health care is one of the few professions where it is socially acceptable to ignore your family, your nonwork life, *yourself.* Gabbard
and Menninger theorized many years ago with respect to physicians as
to why this is so:

> The demands of practice are a convenient rationalization. Phy-
> sicians work long hours to deny dependency, to eradicate any
> trace of aggression or destructiveness that they fear others may
> suspect; win the unconditional love and approval of colleagues,
> patients, and community; to maintain complete control; and to
> conquer the terror of death. It is not the demands of practice,
> but the physicians' compulsive character that wreaks havoc in
> the marriage.[1]

Whether their theory is correct or not, care must be taken not to be
driven in one's career to the extent that everything else loses value and
accordingly does not receive the attention it should. Although being a
healing professional is a wonderful way to devote oneself, unless care
is taken to ensure that the rest of one's life is fulfilling as well, one's life
becomes too narrow, limited, and eventually distorted. This can have a
negative impact not only on oneself but also on family life and other
interpersonal relations.

In a 2003 interview on physician stress, psychiatrist Thomas Cimonetti notes that in social settings, no matter what the gender of the

physician, nonphysician spouses will often gather and speak about family and other life matters, while the physician spouses wind up together speaking about medicine or hospital politics.[2] This natural gravitation to speaking about work-related issues is a problem in any of the helping professions, so it is not surprising that this would occur in medicine.

In addition to workaholism and narrowing of one's horizon so that outside interests, family, and even self are left out, there is the added problem of denial. Most health care professionals would deal with the dangers of burnout or vicarious posttraumatic stress disorder (PTSD) if they were aware of them. They would also view the elements of stress management in a more respectful and serious manner. Stress management includes basic elements (Table 4-1) of which we are aware at some level but do not really "know" at the level of true commitment. When this is so, people who are in intense helping roles pay for this in terms of psychological and physical health—not to mention the havoc it wreaks in the family and on one's necessary social outlets. If people do not pay for it immediately, they do so eventually. The problem with "eventually" is that as in many psychophysical disorders in which psychological stress produces physical changes over time, the damage done that seems so quiet or reversible initially becomes, after a period of time, more or less permanent. At that point, even when stress is reduced and personal is self-care enriched, the physical harm already incurred will have chronic implications for the rest of one's life.

Another reality that we must deal with is that

> The self is limited. It has only so much energy. If it is not renewed, then depletion will take place. Too often we don't avail ourselves of the type of activities that truly renew us. When this occurs we run a greater risk that we will unnecessarily lose perspective and burn out, which is not only sad for us but for the people we are in a position to help in our circle of family, friends, and coworkers.[3]

Sometimes, however, a rude awakening is required for us to realize how far we have drifted from a balanced life. I certainly can vouch for this personally.

> A number of years ago, a very close friend of mine in his early forties was dying, from brain cancer. He was outrageous and

Table 4.1 The Basics of Stress Management

Physical Health

1. *Sleep:* Without enough sleep the quality of what you do will decrease; rising early requires going to bed at a reasonable hour.
2. *Food:* Eating three light meals, at a reasonable pace, and being mindful of the nutritional value of what you eat is one of the best ways to keep weight down and nourishment and energy up.
3. *Exercise:* Taking a fairly brisk walk each day is a good minimum exercise. Doing it on a consistent basis is better than some irregular or future extensive exercise plan which we fail at and feel guilty about.
4. *Leisure:* Relaxing with your feet up and/or being involved in activities that provide genuine enjoyment are not niceties of physical health. Rather, they are undervalued but essential building blocks to good health. Leisure helps us "flow" with life's joys and problems in a more accepting philosophical way.
5. *Pacing:* Taking a little more time to get to a place makes the trip more relaxing; stopping every hour or hour and a half to get out of the car and stretch on long trips makes them a lot more enjoyable and helps increase stamina. Likewise, taking breaks when you feel the need makes your productivity better. The important lesson here is to use any technique necessary to slow yourself down so you don't rush to the grave missing the scenery in your life along the way.

Psychological Stability

1. *Laughter:* If laughter is good medicine, then surely laughing at yourself is healing. We all tend to take ourselves too seriously. So, doing something about this can significantly reduce unnecessary stress and help improve one's perspective on self and life.
2. *Values:* Know what is important and what isn't; by knowing what you believe to be really important you can choose easily and well between alternatives.
3. *Control:* Be careful to discern between what you can control and what you can't; while worrying about something when it happens is natural, continuing to preoccupy yourself with it is not. When you catch yourself worrying endlessly, tease yourself that you must be "the world's best worrier." Then plan what you can do about it, and let it go. If and when it comes up again; review the process until it lessens or stops. This technique may need a good deal of practice for it to "take root" in your attitude.
4. *Self-Appreciation:* Reflect on what gifts . . . [have been] given you, recall them each day in detail (make a list if you have to on paper), and be grateful for them by promising to nurture and share them—not in a compulsive manner but in a generous way. By this I mean have low expectations that people will respond as you would wish or appreciate your efforts. However, simultaneously still try to maintain high hopes that you can appreciate . . . multiple measures of "success" in your work so you don't miss the good that is occurring before you because of a narrow success-oriented viewpoint. For instance, too often we measure what

(Continued)

Table 4-1 (*Continued*)

we achieve at the end of a process and fail to see or value appropriately all of the good we did along the way.

5. *Involvement . . . Not Over-Involvement:* Be active in what you feel is meaningful (the kind of things you would be pleased to reflect on at the very end of life— not necessarily those things that others might feel are impressive or important). Assertiveness on your part both to volunteer to be involved in what you believe is good and to say no to demands that aren't, is also an essential part of increasing your involvement in stimulating activities and curbing (wherever possible) ones that are personally draining.

6. *Support Group:* Have people in your life who care; contact them frequently by phone and in writing as well as in person. Ideally, among this group should be a variety of psychologically healthy friends who can challenge, support, encourage, teach, and make you laugh.

7. *Escape:* There are times when we should "run away" because facing things directly in all of our relationships all the time would be debilitating. To do this you can use novels, breaks during the day, movies, walks, hobbies (fishing, bicycle riding, etc.).

8. *Be Spontaneous:* A small creative action or change during the day or week can make life much more fun. This is a lot more practical than waiting for a yearly vacation.

9. *Be Careful of Negativity:* Often we hear negative comments like thunder and praise like a whisper. Use self-talk to catch your own negative tendencies (i.e., to see things in black-and-white terms, to exaggerate the negative, to let one negative event contaminate the whole day or week, or to discount other positive events). Then answer these thoughts with more accurate positive ones. For example, if you feel slightly depressed and check your thinking, you may see that because one thing went wrong today, you are saying to yourself that you are really a failure at what you do. By recognizing this exaggeration as nonsense, you can tell yourself more correctly that you made a mistake, not that you are a mistake! Following this, you can then recall successes you have had and bring to mind the faces of those who have been grateful for your presence in their lives. This will show you the face of [love] . . . in the world and help break the back of the strong seamless negative thinking you are under at the time. Remember, negative thinking takes a good deal of energy. Stop it, and a great deal of energy will be freed up for growth and enjoyment.

10. *Check Your Individual Balance in the Areas of:*
    a. stimulation and quiet,
    b. reflection and action,
    c. work and leisure,
    d. self-care and care of others,
    e. self-improvement and patience,
    f. future aspirations and present positive realities,
    g. involvement and detachment.

Source: R. J. Wicks, *Touching the Holy: Ordinariness, Self-Esteem and Friendship.* Notre Dame, IN: AMP, 1992. Used with permission.

we constantly teased one another. Even though he was dying, this did not stop.

He had been living in New York and I hadn't seen much of him in the years since I was the best man at his wedding. When he was hospitalized in Philadelphia to undergo experimental treatment, I visited him. When I came to visit he had already been there for almost two weeks.

When I inquired about his health he shared a summary of his condition, which included loss of short-term memory. So, I said to him: "You mean you can't remember what happened yesterday?" He said: "No."

Then I smiled and said: "So, you don't remember me coming in and sitting here with you each day for five hours for the past two weeks?" He looked at me, hesitated for a second or two, grinned widely, and said . . . well I can't share exactly what he said . . . but we both had a good laugh over it.

One of the things he did surprise me with, though, was a question that really helped me put my activities in perspective. He asked: "What good things are you doing now?" As I started to launch into an obsessive (naturally well-organized) list of my recent academic and professional accomplishments, he interrupted me by saying: "No, not that stuff. I mean what really good things have you done? When have you gone fishing last? What museums have you visited lately? What good movies have you seen in the past month?"

The "good things" he was speaking about the last time I saw him alive were different from the ones I in my arrogant good health thought about. Unfortunately, I have a lot of company in this regard.[4]

Naturally, what makes up a self-care protocol varies from person to person and differs according to our stage of life. As Baker notes:

There are many different ways to practice self-care. No one model exists in terms of definition, meaning, significance, or application. Differences between individuals relate to personal history, gender, and personality, and within-individual differences relate to developmental stage, or changing needs. Such differences influence the substance and process of self-care. For one person at a particular stage of life, self-care might involve maintaining a very active schedule and hiring a housekeeper. For another person, or for the same person at a different stage, self-care might involve considerable amounts of quiet, uncommitted personal time and tending one's own home.[5]

Because such a list needs to be tailored, it is helpful to have a large pool of possibilities from which to choose. Listing a number of them here is designed to spur thinking around what could comprise a self-care protocol in your own case. However, there needs to be a sense that the time we spend on self-care is part of the respect needed to live a life of true joy rather than a compulsive rat race under the guise that my profession demands constant presence if I am to be seen as someone who takes it seriously. And so, knowing which elements you might entertain as part of a self-care protocol and questions to ponder in the overall development of it are both good initial steps in acting upon the need to take responsibility for yourself.

Elements of a Self-Care Protocol

There are basic elements of a self-care protocol that almost everyone needs to renew themselves on an ongoing basis. It really does not require too much to take a step back from our work routine to become refreshed and regain perspective. Some of the basic elements might include the following:

- Quiet walks by yourself
- Time and space for meditation
- Spiritual and recreational reading—including the diaries and biographies of others whom you admire
- Some light exercise . . .
- Opportunities to laugh offered by movies, cheerful friends, etc.
- A hobby such as gardening
- Telephone calls to family and friends who inspire and tease you
- Involvement in projects that renew
- Listening to music you enjoy[6]

Other simple steps at self-care and renewal might include the following:

- Visiting a park or hiking
- Having family or friends over for dinner or evening coffee
- Going to the library or a mega-bookstore to have coffee and a scone and to peruse the magazines
- Shopping for little things that would be fun to have but not cost a lot
- Taking a bath rather than a quick shower
- Daydreaming
- Watching a funny movie or going to a comedy club
- Forming a "dining club" in which you go out once a month for lunch with a friend or sibling
- Sending e-mail to friends
- Listening to a mystery book on tape
- Reading poetry out loud
- Staying in bed later than usual on a day off
- Having a leisurely discussion with your spouse over morning coffee in bed
- Watching an old movie
- Making love with your spouse
- Buying and reading a magazine you have never read before
- Fixing a small garden with bright cheery flowers
- Telephoning someone to whom you have not spoken in ages
- Buying and playing a new disk of a singer or musician you love
- Taking a short walk (without using a Walkman) before and after work and/or during lunchtime
- Visiting a diner and having a cup of tea and a piece of pie
- Going on a weekend retreat at a local spirituality center or a hotel on large grounds so you can take out time to walk, reflect, eat when you want, read as long as you like, and just renew yourself
- Arranging to spend a couple of days by yourself in your own home without family or friends present, just to "putz" around and be alone without a schedule or the needs or agendas of others

- Getting a cheap copybook, and journal each day as a way of unwinding
- Asking yourself: What brings you to life? What enlivens your spirit?[7]

Professionals also have the opportunity for continuing education, research and writing, collaboration with colleagues, mentoring—both receiving and offering it, going on a professional or spiritual mini-retreat, and so on; the list is endless. The important thing is to recognize the need to intentionally and spontaneously put these elements into your schedule so they represent a constant, significant portion of the time you have available each day, week, month, and year.

Alice Domar and Henry Dreher, in their book *Self-Nurture*, which is primarily written for women but is filled with good suggestions for us all, refer to the time available as a "time pie." They suggest that once we prepare our list, we then should see how much time we really allot for what we say we are interested in doing for ourselves.

Domar and Dreher write:

> Now compare your list . . . with your time pie. How much time is indicated on the pie for any of the activities listed? Of course, there may be pastimes on your list that you wouldn't do that frequently, like going to a comedy club. But others, like daydreaming or reading, might ideally be part of a typical day. Do these activities show up on our time pie? Many women who follow this exercise discover that there is *no* time on their pie for any of the . . . items. Others count the time spent on purely joyful activity in minutes rather than hours. This can be a shocking revelation, one that motivates some women to radically transform the way they spend their time.[8]

Questions to Ponder in the Development
of a Self-Care Protocol

Time is a very precious commodity for persons in health care. How we allot it, what takes precedence, and with whom we spend it all say a great deal about us and the way we live our lives. In the words of the Dalai Lama from his book *The Path to Tranquility*, "It is very wrong for people to feel deeply sad when they lose some money, yet when they waste the precious moments of their lives they do not have the slightest feeling of repentance."[9] Yet, waste for a physician, nurse, or allied health professional means the wrong thing. The feeling in some is if I take out time for myself, this leisure period is often not seen as "time well spent." Instead, this leisure is seen as almost wrong given all the demands of sick people or, at the very least, this leisure must be earned by having spent a long rotation without any real break during it. To counter this, one must first explore the options available to develop a self-care protocol that is not a nicety of life but rather a necessary source of constant renewal, so that care for others can be done in a quality fashion.

Once one reviews such a list, then how it is used is crucial. At this point, the challenge that presents itself is: *How do we formulate a protocol that we are likely to use beneficially and regularly rather than in spurts?* To ensure an ongoing systematic program is in place, a number of questions have to be asked of oneself first. This is to avoid the dangers, on the one hand, of being unrealistic in developing a protocol and, on the other, of not being creative and expansive enough. Such questions can also help set the stage for designing a personal self-care protocol (as outlined in Table 4-3 at the end of the chapter). Included among these questions are the following:

- Given the changes in the health care system that have resulted in more patient hours, lower status, greater chance for litigation, generally lower financial reward given the importance of the work, and overall insecurity at many levels, what creative ways have you developed to ensure that you do not lose sight of the wonders of health care and the important role you play in it?
- When someone says "self-care," what image comes to mind? What are the positive and negative aspects of this image? In terms of importance and how realistic it is to develop your own self-care protocol, where do you stand?
- In terms of self-care, what is the difference between professionals in health care and other caregivers? How does self-care differ among physicians, nurses, and allied health professionals?
- How do you balance your time apart by yourself to renew your energy, reflect on your life, and clear your thinking with that time you spend with those who challenge and support you and make you laugh?

- Self-care and self-knowledge go hand in hand. What types of activities (i.e., structured reflection at the end of a day, informal debriefing of oneself during the drive home, journaling, mentoring, therapy, spiritual guidance, reading, etc.) in which you are involved will help you develop a systematic and ongoing analysis of how you are progressing in life?
- What types of exercise (walking, the gym, swimming, exercise machine, etc.) do you enjoy and feel would be realistic for you to be involved in on a regular basis?
- Who is in your circle of friends to provide you with encouragement, challenge, perspective, laughter, and inspiration? What ways do you ensure that you have contact with them?
- The balance between work and leisure, professional time and personal time, varies from person to person. What is the ideal balance for you? What steps have you taken to ensure this balance is kept?
- There is a Russian proverb that says: "When you live next to the cemetery, you can't cry for everyone who dies." Self-care involves not getting pulled into the dramatic emotions, fears, and anger that pervade health care settings. What are the self-care elements that support a healthy sense of detachment?
- Being too conservative or being a procrastinator at one end of the spectrum versus being impulsive or too quick to act in the medical setting at the other end are extremes that can be dangerous. How do you maintain a sense of balance that prevents either extreme end of the spectrum?
- How do you prepare for change, which is such a natural part of the health care setting?
- What is the best way you can balance between stimulation and time in silence and solitude so you do not have constant stimulation on the one hand or isolation and preoccupation with self on the other?
- How do you process "unfinished business" (past events, hurts, fears, failures, lost relationships, etc.) in your life so you have enough energy to deal with the challenges and take in the joys in front of you?
- What do you number among the stable forces in your life that are anchors for your own sense of well-being and self-care?

- In what way do you ensure that your goals are challenging and high but not unrealistic and deflating?
- What self-care steps do you have to take because of your gender or race that others of a different race or gender do not have to do?
- How has your past experience set habits in motion that make self-care a challenge in some ways?
- What self-care steps are more important at this stage of your life than they were at earlier life stages?
- What emotional and physical "red flags" are you aware of that indicate you must take certain self-care steps so as not to burn out, violate boundaries, medicate yourself in unhealthy ways, withdraw when you should not, verbally attack patients or colleagues, or drown yourself in work?
- What do you *already* do in terms of self-care? In each of the following areas, what have you found to be most beneficial: physically, socially, professionally, financially, psychologically, and spiritually?
- What is the next step you need to take in developing your self-care protocol? How do you plan to bring this about?
- Are your holidays and vacations appropriately spaced and sufficient for your needs? What is the most renewing way for you to spend this time?
- Are you also conscious of the need for "daily holidays" involving a brief tea or coffee break, a short walk, playing with the children in the evening, or visiting one's friends or parents? Practicing a putt in one's office or living room, practicing a cast with a fly rod in a neighborhood field?

Responding to all of these questions can improve self-knowledge in ways that aid in burnout prevention. They also can increase sensitivity to how you live your life in a way that enables you to both flourish personally and become more faithful and passionate professionally. Once again, the way one moves through the day depends a great deal on personality style. *Burnout is not due to the amount of work but to how we perceive it and interact with people as we do it.* Some people complain that they are so busy that they do not have time to breathe. Others with the same schedule intensity reflect on how happy they are that they are involved in so many challenging projects. All, on the other hand, would complain about the amount of paperwork and documentation that are necessary in modern health care.

Some of us love exercise and thrive on it. Others are more sedentary in their existence. All of us, though, want to be physically healthy.

Not everyone likes outdoor activities and vacations packed with touring new sites and experiencing adventures in different parts of the country or world. Some of us prefer the back yard, a leisurely walk, an artist's easel, a fishing pole, or a good book and a familiar restaurant. However, all of us like to have time away at different points.

The differences among us are many. That is why each self-care protocol, if it is to be both realistic and effective, is unique in its development. The important point is that we must have one in place that we use as a guide every day and not use rationalizations and excuses for not doing this. Not to have a personal self-care protocol is not only courting disaster in terms of both one's personal and professional lives; it is also, at its core, an act of profound disrespect for yourself.

As we learn in our work with patients, bedside manner is an important element of the care for others. I would go even further to say that from a psychological vantage point, respect for them in itself can be transformative. The following illustration with one of my psychotherapy patients illustrates this well. I had seen her for a number of years. She had been sexually abused as a child, and I was seeing her as an adult. We were at the end of a long-term therapy relationship. She had made incredible strides. Her confidence had grown. She was now no longer mired in the past, she had great enthusiasm, and she was one of the most creative persons I had ever met. As we reached the halfway point in the session, I thought it would be a good time to intervene, have her take credit for how far she had come, and get her to reflect on how she had reached this point so that when she entered darkness once again (because darkness comes and goes for everyone who cares), she would know what to do. At least that was my plan. However, it was to end up with a simple surprise . . . for *me*.

> With this plan in mind, . . . I stopped . . . looked at her, and said, "Let's stop for a moment. I have a couple of questions."
>
> She was in the middle of a story, so she was a bit surprised but did as I asked and responded, "What are they?"

"Picture my eyes as a mirror. As you look at them, what do you see?"

She smiled radiantly, showing that she would enjoy this exercise, and said, "I see a person filled with great life. Someone who is excited that she is finally able to find the joyous little girl in herself who had been there before but was lost due to abuse. She has now combined that child with the full grown woman she is now." Then, after a pause, she added with a big smile, "*And*, she is thoroughly happy about it all!"

"Yes." I told her. "That's what I see, too. Given this, the second question I have for you is how did you get to this point? When you first came to see me, you weren't in this place."

My expectation was that she would provide a fairly detailed review of the concrete steps that she took to change her way of viewing herself and the world. Instead, she made a half frown, looked straight at me with her dark brown eyes and said, "You mean you really don't know?"

Taken a bit off guard, I responded, "No. I really don't exactly know."

"Well, it was easy." She said.

> *When I first came to see you,*
> *I simply watched the way you sat with me.*
> *Then I began sitting with myself in the same way.*

For a while I was silent. I had forgotten how a respectful presence to others could be so truly transformative. Such a gentle way of being with others opens up possibilities that are not there when they are able to view themselves only in narrow, unnecessarily negative and distorted ways.[10]

The same can be said of our relationship with ourselves. When we have true self-respect that is evidenced by a sound self-care protocol, it can be transformative for us. As has been alluded to elsewhere in this book, one of the greatest gifts we can share with our coworkers and patients is a sense of our own peace and self-respect. However, you cannot share what you do not have.

Also, we need to recognize that when we speak about self-care and self-nurturing, we are not referring to another intense program that just adds more stress to your life in the name of reducing it. Once again, as Domar and Dreher note:

> True body-nurture absolutely includes physical activity and sound nutrition but not compulsive exercise and onerous dietary restriction. True body-nurture is also much more than exercise and nutrition. It includes the following actions and ideas:
> - Deep diaphragmatic breathing
> - A regular practice of relaxation
> - Cognitive restructuring of body-punishing thoughts into thoughts of compassion and forgiveness
> - Delight in the sensual and sexual pleasures of the body
> - A sane, balanced, non–shame-based relationship with food
> - Health-promoting behaviors, such as stopping smoking, use of alcohol only in moderation, and regular visits to the physician for preventive care
> - A profound regard for the sacredness of the body, including all of its functions, imperfections, idiosyncrasies, and wonders.[11]

Such an overall approach to body-nurture and the other approaches mentioned thus far will clearly benefit us and help us develop an attitude and behaviors that will improve health and increase personal and professional well-being. Before closing this brief treatment of the topic of self-care, I would also like to address the topics of "toxic work" and time management and discuss one particular element of a self-care protocol (reading) that I believe is especially important, to provide a model of how you can take each part of a self-care protocol and personally develop it more deeply as a way of seeing how it can support and challenge you. Finally, I provide a questionnaire designed to aid in the development of one's self-care protocol (Table 4-3) given what has been covered in this chapter. Completing it will provide a summary of the contents of this chapter and a succinct illustration of what the reader believes is involved in self-care for himself or herself.

Toxic Work

In her book *Toxic Work*, Barbara Bailey Reinhold notes:

> The syndrome of toxic work overtakes you when what's happening to you at work causes protracted bouts of distress, cul-

minating in emotional suffering or physical symptoms and heightened by the perceived inability to stop the pain and move on to find or create a more rewarding situation. Feeling stuck where you are, unable to imagine or take your next steps, is perhaps the most debilitating part of the problem.[12]

She also points out that this level of psychological "toxicity" is not going to get better in the near future and that we can

expect more pressure, greater demands, and fewer people employed on-site to do the work. . . . Cost-cutting will be the official support of most organizations both for-profits and nonprofits; budgets will run very close to the wire. . . . Uncertainty will prevail. The only thing you can count on is your own ability to land on your feet when you get knocked off balance by a shift in policy or practice. . . . Increasingly, work will be done primarily in teams. . . . Constant learning will be required particularly in technology [and] . . . you'll need to take responsibility for choreographing your own career and underwriting your own retirement; formerly paternalistic organizations have gotten out of the business of taking care of people.[13]

This sounds very much like what is going on today in modern health care, and responding to it with a sense of negativity or being nostalgic for the "good old days," whereas understandable, will not carry us today. Again, in the words of the author of *Toxic Work*:

Marjorie, a nurse in the day-surgery unit, told me, "We can't wait for this time of cost-cutting to be over, so we can go back to practicing the way we were trained. . . . She belonged to a cadre of "good old days" complainers who gathered in the hospital snack bar at break time each morning.

Fortunately, Marjorie had a friend in pediatrics who had stopped going to the "bitch and moan" sessions, as she called them, because she believed they made things worse. . . . "These are the new policies, and they're not going away," she told Marjorie, "so why don't we go to the hospital fitness room together tomorrow and ride the stationary bikes instead?" Marjorie tried it, was shocked at how different it made her feel. . . .[14]

What Reinhold is pointing out is that if you or other staff members are having a difficult time letting go of percepts of what was in the past, then this is, in her description, a toxic situation that requires health actions.

Such healthy actions include the elements of a self-care protocol thus far included in this chapter, an awareness of the toxic factors that cause stress (noted in chapter 1), a good sense of ourselves so we can be healthy and flexible enough to deal with a constantly changing environment (as was covered in chapter 2), and a willingness to draw from the spiritual wisdom in the world so we can strengthen our inner lives through friendship, community, and those activities that have renewed people through the centuries (as discussed in chapter 3). In addition, we will find in all books addressing the toxic work environment a need to be aware of how we organize and manage our time.

Time Management

An essential part of self-care is being respectful of the limited time we have available during the day. Each person in the health care team needs to have some level of awareness of this area so energy is not unduly wasted. For instance, emergency medical services (EMS) personnel are advised as follows:

1. *Schedule personal time in each day*: Alone time allocated for exercise, meditation, a hobby, or some activity is crucial to the quality of your personal and professional life.
2. *Delegate*: When appropriate at work or home, learn to delegate responsibilities. When you delegate, explain instructions clearly, assign a completion time or date with each task, and follow up once the task is completed. Give positive feedback when appropriate.
3. *Schedule interruptions*: Learn to be flexible in your schedule and off-the-job plans if the telephone rings while you're at home.
4. *Organize*: You can save precious time if you have a designated place for IV catheters, IV fluids, fire hose nozzles, and other such equipment and keep these items where they belong.
5. *Access your resources*: Learn what resources are available to help you do what needs to be done. Learn where these resources are and when you can use them.

6. *Learn to recognize your physical and mental limitations*: Learn *how* and *when* to say no (e.g., "I'm sorry, but I simply don't have time"). Be gentle but firm.[15]

Time management is not a control of time. Rather, it is your ability to use your time more efficiently when personal responsibilities accumulate. Time management techniques themselves can be stressful if careful planning and flexibility are not built into the process.

In his eminently practical book *The Successful Physician*, Marshall Zaslove also includes a discussion of a number of ways physicians—and I believe other health care professionals, too—can improve their productivity. His belief is that just working harder and longer is not the solution. Given this, in this book some of the ideas and recommendations he believes would be beneficial for reflection and discussion with one's colleagues/mentor on the part of physicians (and I believe other health care professionals) are as follows:

- We are not as efficient as we think we are and must start managing ourselves and our careers if we are to be more effective.
- Professional goals provide a psychological rudder, offer us something to focus on and look forward to, help us set priorities, and measure our progress in what are our achievements.
- Looking at areas where time is wasted and doing what you can to prune what is unnecessary will lead to a schedule that is professionally richer and more personally satisfying.
- One of the most costly time wasters is interruptions—seek to limit them with assertiveness and clear feedback to those around you.
- Find your own natural rhythm and work with it.
- Be as attentive as you can when focusing on patients and their problems.
- Design your own ongoing professional education to meet your personal needs.
- Use methods that save time (skim articles, etc.) and integrate knowledge as it relates to actual cases so learning is tailored to the type of cases you are handling rather than simply general or theoretical in nature.
- Have your own panel of experts and knowledge network so you can better learn from your own and others' errors.

- Use an approach that enables you to learn a new procedure in the most effective, least stressful way possible (Table 4-2).

With just a little attention to organization and productivity approaches, so much stress could be reduced. However, often little is done in this area. The feeling may be that this is the kind of information important for people in business or that it is beneath the level of a professional in health care. Obviously, though, when we think of how this would improve patient care and collegiality and enrich the personal life of the nurse, physician, and allied health professional, such views are out of touch with their multifaceted demanding life.

Similarly, not to develop a self-care protocol is also foolish and dangerous—because one of the greatest gifts we can share with our patients is a sense of our own peace, confidence, and energy. Likewise, each element in such a protocol is worth delving into and developing

Table 4-2 How to Learn a New Procedure Faster

With so many new or improved technologies, drug protocols, treatment modalities, and surgical techniques for physicians to learn how to use, there has been more pressure to discover how we can learn a new procedure in the shortest possible time. Here is a brief summary of what seems to work for many physicians:

1. Commit yourself psychologically to learning the new technique . . .
2. If possible, find a highly skilled practitioner to imitate. Make sure she's someone who will slow down, explain the reasons for what she's doing, and take the time to critique you as she checks you out on the procedure . . .
3. Have training sessions in private to avoid embarrassment, especially if you're rusty at basic technique . . .
4. Grasp the sequential steps first by analyzing the procedure intellectually (self-talk helps).
5. Practice individual sub-units of the procedure until you've fixed each one in your mind (chipping) . . .
6. Practice the whole procedure on your own over and over, to gain speed, smoothness, and proficiency.
7. When you're ready, use the new skills as soon and as often as possible in your daily practice.
8. Don't become discouraged by poor outcomes at first. Most procedures take several (even several dozen) reps for basic proficiency, hundreds for mastery.
9. Be prepared to work hard. If it's been some years since you were in training, you may have forgotten the brain-sweat, curses, gritted teeth, and repeated failures of those years.[16]

as completely as possible. To illustrate what I mean by this, I offer the example below of how reading—if thought of in the proper vein—can truly support, challenge, and offer us a new sense of perspective with respect to both our personal and professional life.

Reading

Once, peace activist Dorothy Day was sitting conversing with a homeless alcoholic woman. The woman confessed to Ms. Day that one of the steps she had to take to remain sober was to close her eyes when passing a bar. In response, Dorothy Day said with a commiserating smile, "I know what you mean. I have to do the same thing when I pass a bookstore."

With the publication of the Harry Potter novels, many children who did not read longer books began joyfully jumping into them. Mega-bookstores with cafes that are open late now attract people and tempt them with magazines and books. Yet, many of us still do not read enough. One excuse for this is a seeming lack of time or energy to do so. However, reading—professional or otherwise—can provide new perspectives that may instill new energy and helpful contexts and—in the end—save wasted preoccupation or avoid unnecessary drains on our resources.

Once when I felt on the edge of burnout myself, I thought it was the burden of a very full schedule of teaching, hospital rounds, and patient care that was responsible. On top of this, I was then asked to give a workshop that would require me to research a topic with which I was only marginally familiar. My initial reaction was: "Not yet *another* task to do!" Surprisingly though, when I started reviewing the material for the lecture, I found that the emotional cloud over me was lifting, and I experienced a renewed sense of commitment to what I was already doing. I realized again why I had entered my profession in the first place.

Upon reflection, I realized what had been happening to me. In the day-to-day activities of my work, I had lost the sense of overall intrigue, challenge, and reward that I originally had. I returned to my love of understanding why people behaved the way they did, how a careful analysis of signs and symptoms could point to a better sense of what etiology was at play, what behavioral syndrome might be in play, and how and where one might then profitably place both my and the patient's energies to incur improvement. Professional continuing education, research, and reading were not just additional chores but represented a lifeline to perspective and passion. Reading, and the nourishment it offers us, goes well beyond professional material, as important as that is. We must take steps to improve our overall style of reading as part of a comprehensive approach to self-care.

> Years ago when I was an undergraduate student, the chairperson of the philosophy department and I discussed various interests. Once, when the topic of reading fiction came up, he said that he set aside twenty minutes each night for reading a novel. To this statement I made a facial expression which gave him the message: "Is that all the fiction you read?" In response to my look, he said: "Twenty minutes each night on a regular basis is a heck of a lot of fiction over the period of a year, Bob." And, of course, he was right.

> The important first element in having a reading plan for ourselves so that our hearts are nourished by the ideas, themes, challenges, and hopes of others is for us to set up *regular times to read* to which we will be faithful. Once this is done, we can then address two other issues in developing a reading plan. They are *breadth* and *depth*.

Breadth and Depth

> Even persons who read a great deal still run the risk of getting caught in a rut. Some of us may only read certain types of novels, a particular type of devotional material, or solely material of a certain genre. Just as in the case of our physical well-being, our spiritual health depends upon a varied and balanced "diet" of good reading. Such a diet should include good fiction, autobiographies/biographies, journals, general non-fiction, books of quotations, poetry . . . books of contemporary and "classic" spirituality, and of course sacred scripture.

> *Good Fiction*   In addition to the type of novels we normally enjoy, reading other types of books which challenge and open us up is a good idea. The best-seller list is not the only source of ideas for such reading—as a matter of fact, today it may even be misleading! Winners of the Booker Prize, the Pulitzer, and the National Book Award, as well as suggestions from good friends,

might be better sources. The question "What good books have you read recently?" is a good one to ask of friends whose taste and commitment to a life of meaning you respect.

Autobiographies/Biographies   In the introduction to The Radcliffe Biography Series, Matina S. Horner writes: "Fine biographies give us both a glimpse of ourselves and a reflection of the human spirit. Biography illuminates history, inspires by example, and fires the imagination to life's possibilities. Good biography can create lifelong models for us. Reading about other people's experiences encourages us to persist, to face hardship, and to feel less alone. Biography tells us about choice, the power of a personal vision, and the interdependence of human life."

Reading contemporary autobiographies such as Maya Angelou's *I Know Why the Caged Bird Sings* (Bantam, 1971), Etty Hillesum's *An Interrupted Life* (Pocket Books, 1985), the Dalai Lama's *Freedom in Exile* (Harper, 1991), or Thomas Merton's *Seven Storey Mountain* (Harcourt, Brace and Jovanovich, 1948) all bear out Dr. Horner's comments. Also, reading biographies such as Robert Cole's *Dorothy Day: A Radical Devotion* (Addison-Wesley, 1987) or A.N. Wilson's *C.S. Lewis: A Biography* (Norton, 1990) brings us into the world of persons who can help us see life differently than we might, given our own limited background. The possibilities of both autobiographies and biographies, contemporary and classic, are often overlooked by many of us for more "attractive, exciting reading." Once exposed to this type of book, though, we begin to see that real adventure is entering deeply into the life of another—especially one who faced the despair of life and didn't give in to the situation.

Journals are another way to follow the movements and nuances of people's lives. They, like biographies, also can be quite nourishing and challenging to our souls. Dag Hammarskjold's *Markings* (Knopf, 1976), Kathleen Norris' *Dakota* (Houghton-Mifflin, 1992), Henri Nouwen's *The Genesee Diary* (Doubleday, 1981), and Thomas Merton's *A Vow of Conversation* (Farrar, Straus, and Giroux, 1993) put us in a place where we can explore, piece by piece, the thinking and reactions of individuals trying to make spiritual sense out of the daily occurrences of their lives.

Diaries help us to travel through a geography of reflection which can serve only to help deepen our own sense of healthy introspection. In addition, as we view the diaries of others, their quality of self-understanding can help us move away from morbid and mundane preoccupation with self. They can inspire us to reach out to the world instead of being drawn into a secure quietistic shell of moody self-involvement.

Books of Quotes/Short Reflections   In New York City years ago there were several wonderful authentic Swedish smorgasbords. I just loved them. Such variety! Such quality samplings! Now they are gone, and the brutal buffets of so-so samplings have replaced them throughout the city. As a matter of fact, unfortunately, such blah buffets are everywhere.

A similar scene can be observed with books of quotes. They have proliferated as people seek more and more easy ways to nourish themselves emotionally and spiritually. As a result, motivations regarding why one is seeking such a collection is an important factor in gathering up a volume of quotes for reflection.

If the goal is to sustain oneself on such volumes, then no matter how good a choice made, one's spiritual life will be kept fairly superficial by the use of them. Yet, if books of this type are used as a way to sample wide varieties of hearts and minds and to supplement a regular reading regimen, the results can be quite wonderfully beneficial.

Selection of the type of collection is obviously as important as the place enjoying such material plays in one's reading habits. There are many superb collections of quotes/short reflections available for our use. Anthony de Mello's *One Minute Wisdom* (Doubleday, 1986) Carolyn Warner's *The Last Word* (Prentice-Hall, 1992) and *The Great Thoughts* compiled by George Seldes (Bantam, 1985) are only three that quickly come to mind, but of course there are many more. So, spending a few minutes in a bookstore skimming through selections that initially seem of interest is always a good idea before deciding on which one to buy.

Poetry Books   Most of us read only a line or two of poetry every now and then in a magazine. However, the poetry of such persons as Rilke, Yeats, Frost, or e.e. cummings can break through our fixed ways of viewing life.

Poets see life in such a pristine way that we can be borne up by them to a vantage point we might never see if it weren't for their use of language and meter. . . .

Spirituality Books Volumes specifically designed to help us gain a deeper understanding of our connection to what and Who is greater than our own lives are obviously important as well. Known contemporary writers such as Thomas Merton, Henri Nouwen, Joyce Rupp, James Finley, Kathleen Fischer, Metropolitan Anthony of Sourozh (Anthony Bloom), Gerald May, William Barry, Abraham Heschel, and Basil Pennington are good to sample. In addition the classic works . . . such as *The Cloud of Unknowing* and *Way of the Pilgrim* are also good sources. [If you are Christian] moving beyond one's own tradition to read from other religious traditions is also very enlightening and inspiring. Examples of this would be the *Tao Te Ching*, the *Kabbalah*, and the many fine works from non-Christian religions available in Paulist Press' Classics of Western Spirituality series.[17]

And so, reading can bring psychological and spiritual nourishment in so many ways *if* we avail ourselves of it in a structured way that involves time, breadth, and depth in our selections. A final suggestion in this area is to include time for reflection on what you have read. I actually underline in the books I read, and I copy out some of those underlined passages if I feel they are truly important to keeping perspective and hope alive within me. Finally, I review the comments several times during the week or month so I can make the lessons they hold a part of the way I live. I have found that the impact of this on those I mentor to be quite impressive.

By taking each element of a self-care protocol and developing it as I have done here, you can create a rich tapestry of activities and approaches to self-understanding and renewal. First, though, it is important to create a sufficiently broad outline of what would comprise the elements of a personally designed self-care protocol given your own needs, work, family life, personality style, and stage of life. To this end, this chapter is concluded by providing a suggested format (Table 4-3) to use as a springboard in the development of what would support, challenge, and give you perspective as you continue on the road in one of the most demanding and rewarding careers one can have: health care.

Table 4-3 Self-Care Protocol Questionnaire

Please note: This material is for your own use. There is a tendency on the part of some to be quick, terse, and often global in their responses. Such defensiveness, although natural, limits the helpfulness of completing this questionnaire to gain as full an awareness as possible of your current profile and the personal goals you plan to develop for a realistic yet appropriately balanced and rich self-care program. Consequently, in preparing this personally designed protocol, the more clear, specific, complete, imaginative, and realistic your responses are to the questions provided, the more useful the material will be in integrating it into your schedule.

1. List healthy *nutritional practices* that you currently have in place.
2. What are specific realistic ways to improve your eating/drinking (of alcoholic beverages) habits?
3. What *physical exercise* do you presently get, and when is it scheduled during the week?
4. What changes do you wish to make in your schedule in terms of time, frequency, and variety with respect to exercise?
5. Where are the periods for reflection, quiet time, meditation, mini-breaks alone, opportunities to center yourself, and personal debriefing times now in your schedule?
6. Given your personality style, family life, and work situation, what changes would you like to make in your schedule to make it more intentional and balanced with respect to processing what comes to the fore in your time spent alone or in silence?
7. How much, what type, and how deeply and broadly do you read at this point?
8. What would you like to do to increase variety or depth in your reading, research, and continuing education pursuits?
9. Below, list the activities present in your nonworking schedule not previously noted here. Along with the frequency/time, list changes to this schedule that you believe would further enrich you personally/professionally as well as have a positive impact, in turn, on your family, colleagues, and overall social network.

Activities Frequency/Time Now Allotted or Planned to Change/Improvement
Leisure time with:
    Spouse/Significant Other
    Children
    Parents
    Family members
    Friends
Going to movies
Watching TV
Visiting museums
Sports
Attending concerts/plays
Listening to music

Hiking, biking, walking, or swimming
Making telephone calls to family and friends
Hobbies (gardening, coin collecting, etc.)
Eating out for dinner
Shopping
Going to libraries, bookstores, coffee shops
Sending e-mail to friends
Making love
Journaling
Continuing education
Vacations
Spending long weekends away
Meditation/reflection/sitting zazen
Religious rituals
Leisurely baths
Massage
Other activities not listed above:

_____
_____
_____
_____

10. What are the ways you process strong emotions (i.e., anger, anxiety, deep sadness, confusion, fear, emotional "highs" or the desire to violate boundaries for reasons of personal/sexual/financial/power gratifications)?
11. Where in your schedule do you regularly undertake such emotional processing?
12. What would you like to do to change the extent and approaches you are now using for self-analysis/debriefing of self?
13. Who comprise the interpersonal anchors in your life?
14. What do you feel is lacking in your network of friends?
15. What are some reasonable initiatives you wish to undertake to have a richer network?
16. What are your sleep/rest habits now?
17. If you are not getting enough sleep/rest, what are some realistic ways to ensure you get more?

Note: This is just a partial questionnaire. Please feel free to include, analyze, and develop a plan for improvement and integration of other aspects of self-care. Also, review your answers at different points to see what resistances to change come up and how you can face them in new creative ways by yourself or with the help of a friend, colleague, mentor, or professional counselor or therapist.

Objectives of Chapter Four

- Recognize the impoverishment of a single-minded devotion to career and nothing else
- Know the basics of stress management in terms of physical health and psychological stability
- Be familiar with the varied elements possible to include in a self-care protocol
- Know the type of questions to pose to yourself and those you mentor as a way to develop a self-care protocol
- Appreciate the role of self-respect in one's attitude as a key determinant in self-care
- Possess an a awareness of the concept "toxic work"
- Be familiar with the key elements of time management

Additional Books to Consider

Marshall Zaslov's book *The Successful Physician* is based on the tenet that we are not as efficient as we think we are and must start managing ourselves and our careers to really be effective. In his book he gives good advice on cutting paperwork, rearranging clinical work, how to update your clinical knowledge in the most efficient ways possible, and ways to improve communication with staff and patients. It is a very helpful and realistic book. Sherry Kahn and Mileva Saulo's *Healing Yourself: A Nurse's Guide to Self-Care and Renewal*, Barbara Reinhold's book *Toxic Work*, Ellen Baker's book for psychologists, *Caring for Ourselves*, and the popular trade book *Self-Nurture: Learning to Care for Yourself as Effectively as You Care for Everyone Else* all contain very useful information for nurses, physicians, and allied health professionals.

Notes

1. G. Gabbard and R. Menninger, *Medical Marriages* (Washington, DC: American Psychiatric Press, 1988), 35.

2. Interview with Thomas Cimonetti (2003).

3. R. Wicks, *Riding the Dragon* (Notre Dame, IN: Sorin Books, 2003), 46.

4. R. Wicks, *After 50: Spiritually Embracing Your Own Wisdom Years* (Mahwah, NJ: Paulist Press, 1997)

5. E. Baker, *Caring for Ourselves* (Washington, DC: American Psychological Association, 2003), 18–19.

6. R. Wicks, Op. Cit (2003), 50.

7. I added this last point as a result of a personal communication with Beverly Eanes. She also notes in the book she wrote with L. Richmond and J. Link, *What Brings You to Life* (Mahwah, NJ: Paulist Press, 80, 81), "We need the freedom to be and the space to receive life. Sometimes like seeds, we need fallow time. Like seeds, we need the time of autumn and winter in order to bud in the spring and flower in summer. It also means that we don't have to feel guilty when we stand and wait, or when we rest."

8. A. Domar and H. Dreher, *Self-Nurture* (New York: Penguin, 2000), 198.

9. Dalai Lama, *The Path to Tranquility* (New York: Viking, 1999), 73.

10. R. Wicks, *Living a Gentle, Passionate Life* (Mahwah, NJ: Paulist Press, 1998), 29, 30.

11. Domar and Dreher, Op. Cit., 99.

12. B. Reinhold, *Toxic Work* (New York: Plume, 1997), 15.

13. Ibid., 34, 25.

14. Ibid., 105.

15. B. Seward, *Managing Stress in Emergency Medical Services* (Sudbury, MA: American Academy of Orthopaedic Surgeons/Jones and Bartlett, 2000), 42.

16. M. Zaslove, *The Successful Physician* (Gaithersburg, MD: Aspen, 1998), 166–168.

17. R. Wicks, Op. Cit. (1997), 63–67.

Passionate Journeys

Returning to the Wonders of Medicine, Nursing, and Allied Health

Physician Albert Schweitzer once said, "I don't know what your destiny will be, but one thing I do know, the only ones among you who will be really happy are those who have sought and found how to serve."[1] Physicians, nurses, and allied health professionals, by their entry and faithfulness to the health care mission, certainly have taken this admonishment to heart. The goal throughout the book you have just read has been to provide direction, information, and encouragement to respect the real dangers incurred to one's psychological and physical health in the process of fulfilling a personal commitment to this intense mission. As was pointed out, in addition to the personal benefit the medical/nursing professional derives from self-care, how one addresses this area can have a beneficial impact on those being served. It is no surprise that unfortunate—and sometimes even fatal—consequences for innocent patients may be attributable to the inattentiveness and exhaustion of harried, hurried health care personnel who ignore or minimize the value of both self-care and self-knowledge.

In the introduction to a special issue of *Medical Encounter* (a publication of the American Academy on Physician and Patient) that was dedicated to physician well-being, Christensen and Suchman sum up this situation quite well:

> Caring for the health of human beings is a vocation that has
> summoned forth some of the noblest and most valued work in

human societies through the millennia. From its origins in shamanism; its later development in theology, philosophy, and science; and in recent decades its evolution from a cottage industry to integrated systems of health care, medicine has served humanity by easing suffering and providing comfort in times of distress, and in recent centuries by extending the human life span and compressing the duration and severity of illness. As professionals currently serving in this enterprise—physicians, nurses, medical assistants, administrators, psychologists, social workers, and others—we are privileged to participate in an epic human endeavor. We are also at high risk of overwork, burnout, and more serious impairment.

With increased integration of services, constraints on society's financing of health care, a swelling of the population moving into advanced age, and the acceleration of information processing technologies—increased demands are falling on the backs of professionals throughout the healthcare spectrum for increased productivity, documentation, vigilance to prevent error, and mastery of expanding areas of knowledge and technology. We often find ourselves racing to keep up with all our tasks without having time to reflect on the deeper meaning of our vocation. The load we are carrying increasingly exceeds our carrying capacity.[2]

Yet, even though the realistic strains of modern health care are great, the theme and philosophical stance of this book have been that *recapturing the awe of being a physician, nurse, or allied health professional is within reach with some knowledge and action.* What is almost lost can be rediscovered. What is presently possessed need not be given away. A recently graduated nurse at a leading teaching hospital shared with me how much joy her work was bringing her. In doing this, she then described some of her cases and challenges, as well as her frustrations. Chief among her complaints was that some of her co-workers in the intensive care unit where she worked seemed drained, jaded, and unmotivated. She said in a hoarse voice, "I don't want to be like them. Nursing is a gift I don't want to lose or take for granted." My point in writing this book is that she does not have to be like her co-workers.

This book then has been about retaining and deepening the gift of passion for the care of others while realistically facing the interior and systemic problems that are part of an involved life—especially in such personally and intellectually demanding fields as medicine, nursing, and allied health. It has also dealt with having a real sensitivity to the acute and chronic dangers to one's health while not consequently forsaking the honor and privilege of working in medicine and nursing. In addition, and of equal importance, it has been about diagnosing the problems of secondary stress early, taking action—both preventive and ameliorative—as soon as possible, and reviewing the results of such ongoing interventions. To do this, one has to be aware of what can be learned from the literature on the topic and from clinical work with people involved in health care today. Above all, it is about coming home to oneself in a way that self-knowledge, strengthening one's inner life, and self-care are not considered "a given" or "a luxury" but are instead intentionally embraced as part of an essential ongoing process. Such a process, like good medicine, produces good results and a return to the wonder and awe that entering and remaining in the medical, nursing, and allied health fields can and should produce.

There is a need for an ongoing monitoring of oneself and a continual posing of questions such as the following:

> What approaches are most helpful for me to take to deal with the systemic and personal stresses in my life?
> What additional knowledge/support do I need to take actions to accomplish a better program of self-care and increased self-knowledge?
> How can I strengthen my inner life so I can have a richer personal and professional life?

In the previous four chapters, I enumerated the many benefits of facing these questions in a conscious, ongoing (sometimes formal) way. To review, some of the primary benefits include:

- An ability to focus on the patient in front of you—no matter how full your day may be
- Having a sense of intrigue about your talents and growing edges in a way that helps you deepen both as a professional and as a person
- A willingness and facility to appropriately handle strong emotions, deal with different patients/colleagues, clarify

roles, and improve your level of satisfaction in interpersonal relations
- A recognition of the need for time apart to reflect, reassess, and replenish yourself
- Awareness of the signs of chronic irritability, fatigue, constant daydreaming, greater effort with lesser job satisfaction, inability to relax, and a tendency to be preoccupied with work as warnings that chronic secondary stress needs to be limited before it becomes too severe

Naturally, the tables, content of the chapters, and recommended further reading contain even greater information on this. Reviewing the text and your responses to the questionnaires provided will enable you to make a summary of the material that is tailored to you.

The Joys of Medicine, Nursing, and Allied Health

As one takes reasonable steps toward facing the challenges of *secondary* stress, to retain a sense of perspective there is also a need to recall the joys of being a professional in health care today. Too often we focus on just the dangers, challenges, and stress, and we fail to recall the joys. Being a nurse, physician, or allied health professional is very rewarding in so many ways. These include:

- An opportunity to save, improve, or prolong people's lives
- Receiving the trust and being part of the dramatic elements of peoples' lives not open to many other people/professionals
- Being part of a field whose knowledge base is dynamic and deep
- Having the security of knowing medical/nursing professionals will always be needed and valued
- Experiencing a sense of potency because of the impact you may have on other peoples' lives
- Being given the opportunity to interact with a wide range of people and emotions in a myriad of situations
- Being in a position to be both intrigued and challenged by the resistance of a disease (and sometimes the person carrying it!) to the treatment protocol you provide

- Knowing firsthand the benefit of both good organization and creativity in providing sound treatment—and the challenges that lie in knowing when one takes precedent over the other
- Appreciating the essential role your own personality, spirituality, and psychological health has in delivering effective health care
- Having the chance to be a "medical detective" as you seek to uncover what symptoms and signs mean as you track and/or unmask a previously undiagnosed/undetected disease or illness in a patient

The joys or job satisfaction can be so great. However, as in the case of self-care, they are not a given. They must be appreciated and attended to in our lives. As Lachman[3] points out in her book on nursing and stress management, there is a need to raise our awareness of what the elements in job satisfaction are so we can turn the tide in favor of progress over the status quo.

There are several other variables that contribute to your job satisfaction. By focusing specifically on a few, you could turn the tide of your disappointment in your present job or even in nursing in general... .

- *Workload.* Believe it or not, some nurses complain of too little work and feel bored! Most of you are on the opposite end of the continuum, complaining of overload...
- *Physical variables.* Temperature, humidity, little or no light, noise, and chemicals are all factors affecting your physical environment.
- *Job status.* A low or negative social status creates psychological discomfort.
- *Accountability.* This is the extent to which important outcomes depend on your performance in relation to the amount of control you have over the results.
- *Task variety.* Is your task variety balanced so that you are satisfied with this variable?
- *Human contact.* Occasionally administrators and/or nurses complain about too little human contact. However, most nurses have desert island fantasies by the end of the day because they are so stimulated by people overload... . Do you want more or less human contact, or are you satisfied?

- *Physical challenge.* How much dexterity, physical skill or strength, endurance, or physical mobility do you need on your job? If you are a highly physical person and your job has little activity, you are likely to experience some degree of frustration.... Perhaps you are not a physical person and this little activity is satisfying for you at work. Be kind to your body and moderately exercise after work, especially if your job is sedentary.
- *Mental challenge.* People perform better if they use their cognitive skills to some degree. These skills include observing, recognizing, memorizing, monitoring, comparing, evaluating, deciding, and reasoning.[3]

In an article on physician satisfaction, similar sentiments are noted. One of the particular points made is that

> higher perceived stress is associated with lower satisfaction levels that are related to greater intentions to quit, decrease work hours, change specialty, or leave direct patient care. One can see here the powerful effect of the combination of job stress and dissatisfaction. So powerful, in fact, that some of these highly trained, committed professionals may leave their practice situations while others cope by decreasing work hours, changing practice emphasis or leaving direct patient care.[4]

When faced with stress, physicians, nurses, and allied health professionals all act. The question this book confronts is: How do we act? If we do not develop careful strategies, either inactivity or unhealthy actions will certainly fill the void. It is my hope in writing this book that the reader will set aside resistance that claims that approaches to understanding, limiting, and overcoming secondary stress are unrealistic. After reading this book, using the questionnaires and tables as follow-up, and revisiting the book when issues come up again—and they will—I believe that the practitioners will be able to navigate the waves of stress that come in health care in the most healthy way possible. Moreover, the result of such experiences will open the physician, nurse, and allied health professional to be a deeper person and a helpful mentor to colleagues who, like them, give much and deserve all the support and wisdom we can share with them.

Notes

1. Statement by Albert Schweitzer cited in *The Way to Happiness* by Gilbert Hay (New York: Simon and Schuster, 1967), 35.

2. J. Christensen and A. Suchman, "Introduction." *Medical Encounter*, 16, 4 (Spring 2002): 2.

3. V. Lachman, *Stress Management: A Manual for Nurses* (New York: Grune and Stratton, 1983), 116.

4. E. Williams, T. Konrad, W. Scheckler, D. Pathman, M. Linzer, J. McMurray, M. Schwartz, and M. Gerrity, "Understanding Physicians' Intentions to Withdraw from Practice: The Role of Job Satisfaction, Job Stress, and Mental and Physical Health," *Health Care Management Review*, 26, 1 (2001): 15.

Bibliography

Aach RD, et al. Stress and Impairment During Residency Training: Strategies for Reduction, Identification, and Management. Annals of Internal Medicine (1988), 154–161.

Aach RD, Girard DE, et al. Alcohol and Other Substance Abuse and Impairment among Physicians in Residency Training. American College of Physicians (1992), Vol. 116:245–254.

Ackerley GD, Burnell J, Holder DC, and Kurdek LA. Burnout among Licensed Psychologists. Professional Psychology: Research and Practice (1988), Vol. 19:624–631.

Adler G. Helplessness in the Helpers. British Journal of Medical Psychology (1972), Vol. 45:315–326.

Adler R, Werner ER, Korsch B. Systematic Study of Four Years of Internship. Pediatrics (1980), Vol. 66:1000–1008.

Agius RM, Blenkin H, Deary IJ, et al. Survey of Perceived Stress and Work Demands of Consultant Doctors. Occupational and Environment Medicine (1996), Vol. 53:217–224.

Albright CL, Winkleby M, Ragland D, Fisher J, and Syme SL. Job Strain and Prevalence of Hypertension in a Biracial Population of Urban Bus Drivers. American Journal of Public Health (1992), Vol. 82:984–989.

Alexander D, Monk JS, and Jonas AP. Occupational Stress, Personal Strain, and Coping Among Residents and Faculty Members. Journal of Medical Education (1985), Vol. 60:830–839.

Allanach EL. Perceived Supportive Behaviors and Nursing Occupational Stress: An Evolution of Consciousness. Advances in Nursing Science (1988), January:73–82.

Allen J and Mellor D. Work Context, Personal Control and Burnout Amongst Nurses. Western Journal of Nursing Research (2002), Vol. 24:905–918.

Alloy LB and Abramson LY. Depressive Realism: Four Theoretical Perspectives. In L Alloy (Ed.), Cognitive Processing in Depression. New York: Guilford Press (1988), 223–265.

Alloy LB and Abramson LY. Learned Helplessness, Depression, and the Illusion of Control. Journal of Personality and Social Psychology (1982), Vol. 36:1114–1126.

Alpern F, Correnti CE, Dolan TE, et al. A Survey of Recovering Maryland Physicians. Maryland Medical Journal (1992), Vol. 41:301–303.

Altun I. Burnout and Nurses' Personal and Professional Values. Nursing Ethics (2002), Vol. 9:3:269–278.

Ammerman RT, Cassisi JE, Hersen M, and Van-Hasselt VB. Consequences of Physical Abuse and Neglect in Children. Clinical Psychology Review (1986), Vol. 6:291–310.

Ankney RN, Coil JA, Kolff J, et al. Physician Understanding of the National Practitioner Data Bank. Southern Medical Journal (1995), Vol. 88:200–203.

Anonymous. Burnished or Burnt Out: The Delights and Dangers of Working in Health. Lancet (1994), Vol. 344:1583–1584.

Arnetz BB. White Collar Stress: What Studies of Physicians Can Teach Us. Psychotherapy and Psychosomatics (1991), Vol. 55:197–200.

Aschenbrener CA and Siders CT. Managing Low-to-Mid Intensity Conflict in the Health Care Setting. The Physician Executive (1999), Vol. 25:44–50.

Asken MJ and Raham DC. Resident Performance and Sleep Deprivation: A Review. Journal of Medical Education (1983), Vol. 58:382–387.

Auden WH. Introduction to Dag Hammarskjold's Markings. New York: Knopf (1976), ix.

Bacharach S and Mitchell S. The Quality of Working Life of Professional, Technical, and Scientific Employees of New York State. Report to the Joint Labor-Management Committee on Professional Development and QWL, NYSSILR. Ithaca, NY: Cornell University (1982).

Bacharach SB, Bamberger P, and Conley, S. Work-Home Conflict among Nurses and Engineers: Mediating the Impact of Role Stress on Burnout and Satisfaction at Work. Journal of Organizational Behavior (1991), Vol. 12:39–53.

Bailey JT. Stress and Stress Management: An Overview. Journal of Nursing Education (1980), Vol. 19:5–7.

Bailey R and Clarke M. Stress and Coping in Nursing. New York: Chapman and Hall (1989).

Baker E. Caring for Ourselves: A Therapist's Guide to Personal and Professional Well-being. Washington, DC: American Psychological Association (2003).

Baldwin DC, Hughes PH, Conrad SE, et al. Substance Use among Senior Medical Students: A Survey of 23 Medical Schools. Journal of the American Medical Association (1991), Vol. 265:2074–2078.

Baldwin PJ, Dodd M, and Wrate RW. Young Doctors' Health, I. How Do Working Conditions Affect Attitudes, Health and Performance? Social Science and Medicine (1997), Vol. 45:35–40.

Balon R, Mufti R, Williams M, and Riba M. Possible Discrimination in Recruitment of Psychiatry Residents. American Journal of Psychiatry (1997), Vol. 154:11:1608–1609.

Barnum B. Spirituality in Nursing, 2nd Edition: From Traditional to New Age. New York: Springer (2003).

Baron RA. Understanding Human Relations: A Practical Guide to People at Work. Boston, MA: Allyn and Bacon (1985).

Bates EM and Moore BN. Stress in Hospital Personnel. Medical Journal of Australia (1975), Vol. 2:765–767.

Beaumier A, Bordage G, Saucier D, and Turgeon J. Nature of the clinical difficulties of first-year family medicine residents under direct observation. Canadian Medical Association Journal (1992), Vol. 146:489–497.

Beck AT, Steer RA, and Garbin MG. Psychometric Properties of the Beck Depression Inventory: Twenty-five Years of Evaluation. Clinical Psychology Review (1988), Vol. 8:77–100.

Beck DF. Counselor Burnout in Family Service Agencies. Social Casework (1987), January.

Bedeian A and Armenakis A. A Path-Analytic Study of the Consequences of Role Conflict and Ambiguity. Academy of Management Journal (1981), Vol. 24:417–424.

Beehr TA. The Role of Social Support in Coping with Organizational Stress. In TA Beehr and RS Bhagat (Eds.), Human Stress and Condition in Organizations: An Integrated Perspective. New York: John Wiley and Sons (1985), 375–398.

Beehr TA and McGrath JE. Social Support, Occupational Stress and Anxiety. Anxiety, Stress and Coping (1992), Vol. 5:7–19.

Beehr TA and Newman JE. Job Stress, Employee Health, and Organizational Effectiveness: A Facet Analysis, Model, and Literature Review. Personality Psychology (1978), Vol. 31:665–699.

Bennett G. Faculty Interventions: How Far Should You Go? In CD Scott and J Hawk (Eds.), Heal Thyself: The Health of Health Care Professionals. New York: Brunner Mazel Publishers (1986), 147–160.

Ben-Sira Z. Affective and Instrumental Components in the Physician-Patient Relationship: An Additional Dimension of Interaction Theory. Journal of Health and Social Behavior (1980), Vol. 21:170–180.

Ben-Sira Z. Chronic Illness, Stress and Coping. Social Science and Medicine (1984),Vol. 16:1013–1019.

Ben-Sira Z. Involvement with a Disease and Primary Care Utilization. Sociology of Health and Illness (1980),Vol. 2:247–276.

Ben-Sira Z. Lay Evaluation of Medical Treatment and Competence: Development of a Model of the Function of the Physician's Affective Behavior. Social Science and Medicine (1982),Vol. 16:1013–1019.

Ben-Sira Z. Primary Medical Care and Coping with Stress and Disease: The Inclination of Primary Care Practitioners to Demonstrate Affective Behavior. Social Science and Medicine (1985),Vol. 21:5:485–498.

Ben-Sira Z. Societal Integration of the Disabled: Power Struggle or Enhancement of Individual Coping Capacities. Social Science and Medicine (1985), Vol. 17:1011–1014.

Ben-Sira Z. Stress and Illness: A Revised Application of the Stressful Life Events Approach Research Communications in Psychology, Psychiatry and Behavior (1981),Vol. 6:317–327.

Berg JK. One Hundred Alcoholic Women in Medicine: An Interview Study. Journal of American Medical Association (1987),Vol. 55:851–857.

Berg JK and Garrad J. Psychosocial Support in Residency Training Programs. Journal of Medical Education (1980),Vol. 55:851–857.

Bergman AS. Marital Stress and Medical Training: An Experience with a Support Group for Medical House Staff Wives. Pediatrics (1980),Vol. 65:944–947.

Bjorksten O, Sutherland S, Miller C, and Stewart T. Identification of Medical Student Problems and Comparison with Those of Other Students. Journal of Medical Education (1983),Vol. 58:759–767.

Blachly PH, Disher W, and Roduner G. Suicide by Physicians. Bulletin of Suicidology, National Institute of Mental Health, pp 1–18, December 1968.

Blackwell B. Prevention of Impairment among Residents in Training. Journal of American Medical Association (1986),Vol. 255:9:1177–1178.

Blackwell B, Gutmann M, and Jewell K. Role Adoption in Residency Training. General Hospital Psychiatry (1984),Vol. 6:280–288.

Block D. Foreword in Heal Thyself: The Health of Health Care Professionals. In C Scott and J Hawk (Eds.), New York: Brunner Mazel Publishers (1986), ix.

Bloom A. Beginning to Pray. Ramsey, NJ: Paulist Press (1970).

Blume SB. Women and Alcohol: A Review. Journal of American Medical Association (1986),Vol. 256:1467–1470.

Bode R. First You Have to Row a Little Boat. New York: Warner (1993), 49.

Bodnar JC and Kiecolt-Glaser JK. Caregiver Depression After Bereavement: Chronic Stress Isn't Over When It's Over. Psychology and Aging (1994), Vol. 9:3:372–380.

Bojar S. Psychiatric Problems of Medical Students. In GB Blain and CC McArthur (Eds.), Emotional Problems of the Student. New York: Appleton-Century-Crofts (1971), 350–363.

Bond M. Stress and Self-Awareness: A Guide for Nurses. Rockville, MD: Aspen Publishers (1986).

Borenstein DB. Job Satisfaction for the Training Years: A New Mental Healthy Program at UCLA. Journal of the American Medical Association (1982), Vol. 247:19:2700–2703.

Borus J. The Transition to Practice. Journal of Medical Education (1971), Vol. 57:593–601.

Boswell CA. Work Stress and Job Satisfaction for the Community Health Nurse. Journal of Community Health Nursing (1992), Vol. 9:221–228.

Bowman GD and Stern M. Adjustment to Occupational Stress: The Relationship of Perceived Control to Effectiveness of Coping Strategies. Journal of Counseling Psychology (1995), Vol. 42:3:194–203.

Boyle BP and Coombs RH. Personality Profiles Related to Emotional Stress in the Initial Year of Medical Training. Journal of Medical Education (1971), Vol. 46:882–888.

Brazier D. Zen Therapy. New York: Wiley (1995).

Brewster JM. Prevalence of Alcohol and Other Drug Problems among Physicians. Journal of the American Medical Association (1986), Vol. 255:1913–1920.

Brief AP, Burke MJ, George JM, Robinson B, and Webster J. Should Negative Affectivity Remain an Unmeasured Variable in the Study of Job-Related Stress? Journal of Applied Psychology (1988), Vol. 73:193–198.

Briere J. Therapy for Adults Molested as Children: Beyond Survival. New York: Springer (1989).

British Medical Association. Stress and the Medical Profession. London: British Medical Association (1992).

Brogan DJ, Frank E, Elon L, Sivanesan SP, and O'Hanlan KA. Harassment of Lesbians as Medical Students and Physicians. Journal of American Medical Association (1999), Vol. 282:13:1290–1292.

Brollier C. Managerial Leadership and Staff OTR Job Satisfaction. Occupational Therapy Journal of Research (1987), Vol. 5:3, 171–184.

Brollier C, Bender D, Cyranowski J, and Velletri CM. A Pilot Study of Job Burnout among Hospital-Based Occupational Therapists. The Occupational Therapy Journal of Research (1988), Vol. 6:5, 285–299.

Brollier C, Bender D, Cyranowski J, and Velletri CM. OTR Burnout: A Comparison by Clinical Practice and Direct Service Time. Occupational Therapy in Mental Health (1987), Vol. 7:1:39–54.

Brown N. Ministerial Burnout and Personality. Unpublished manuscript, Pasadena, CA: Fuller Theological Seminary (1985).

Brown S. The Stresses of Clinical Medicine. In Not Another Guide to Stress in General Practice! (2nd edition). Oxford: Radcliffe Medical Press (2000), 52.

Bryson J, Bryson R, and Johnson M. Family Size, Satisfaction, and Productivity in Dual Career Couples. Psychology of Women Quarterly (1978), Vol. 3:10–16.

Buber M. Way of Man. New York: Lyle Stuart (1966).

Buckley LM, Sanders K, Shih M, and Hampton CL. Attitudes of Clinical Faculty about Career Progress, Career Success and Recognition, and Commitment to Academic Medicine. Archives of Intern Med (2000), Vol. 160. www.archinternmed.com

Bunch WH, Dvonch VM, Storr CL, Baldwin DC, and Hughes PH. The Stresses of the Surgical Residency. Journal of Surgical Research (1992), 53:268–271.

Burke R, Weir T, and Duwors R. Work Demands on Administrators and Spouse Well-being. Human Relations (1980), Vol. 33:253–278.

Burke RJ. Stressful Event, Work-Family Conflict, Coping, Psychological Burnout, and Well-being Among Police Officers. Psychological Reports (1994), Vol. 75:787–800.

Burke RJ and Richardson AM. Sources of Satisfaction and Stress among Canadian Physicians. Psychol Rep (1990), Vol. 67:1335–1344.

Burns D. Feeling Good. New York: Thomas More/Sorin Books (2000).

Butterfield PA. The Stress of Residency. Archives of Internal Medicine (1988), Vol. 148:1428–1435.

Buunk BP and Hoorens V. Social Support and Stress: The Role of Social Comparison and Social Exchange Processes. British Journal of Clinical Psychology (1992), Vol. 31:445–457.

Buunk BP and Schaufeli WB. Professional Burnout: A Perspective from Social Comparison Theory. In WB Schaufeli, C Maslach, and T Marek (Eds.), Professional Burnout: Recent Developments in Theory and Research. New York: Hemisphere (1993), 53–69.

Byrd R. Alone. New York: Putnam (1938); reprinted New York: Kodansha (1995).

Byrne BM. The Maslach Burnout Inventory: Validating Factorial Structure and Invariance Across Intermediate, Secondary, and University Educators. Multivariate Behavioral Research (1991), Vol. 26:4:583–605.

Caldwell T and Weiner MF. Stresses and Coping in ICU Nursing. General Hospital Psychiatry (1981), Vol. 3:199–227.

Callahan EJ, Jaen CR, Crabtree BF, Zyzanski SJ, Goodwin MA, and Strange KC. The Impact of Recent Emotional Distress and Diagnosis of Depression or Anxiety on the Physician-Patient Encounter in Family Practice. Journal of Family Practice (1998), Vol. 46:410–418.

Callan JP (Ed.). The Physician: A Professional Under Stress. Norwalk, CT: Appleton-Century-Crofts (1983).

Capner M and Caltabiano ML. Factors Affecting the Progression Towards Burnout: A Comparison of Professional and Volunteer Counsellors. Psychological Reports (1993), Vol. 73:555–561.

Carnes M. Balancing Family and Career: Advice from the Trenches. Annals of Internal Medicine (1996), Vol. 125:7:618–620.

Cartwright LK. Sources and Effects of Stress in Health Careers. In GC Stone, F Cohen, and NE Adler (Eds.), Health Psychology. San Francisco, Jossey-Bass (1979).

Celentano D and Johnson JV. Stress in Health Care Workers. Occupational Medicine (1987), Vol. 2:593–608.

Ceslowitz SB. Burnout and Coping Strategies among Hospital Staff Nurses. Journal of Advanced Nursing (1989), Vol. 14:553–558.

Chadwick D. The Crooked Cucumber. New York: Broadway (1999).

Chan WC, Sunshine JH, Owen JB, and Shaffer KA. U.S. Radiologists' Satisfaction in Their Profession. Radiology (1995), Vol. 194:649–656.

Cherniss C. Beyond Burnout. New York: Routledge (1995).

Cherniss C. Professional Burnout in Human Service Organizations. New York, Praeger (1980).

Cherniss C. Role of Professional Self-Efficacy in the Etiology and Amelioration of Burnout. In WB Schaufelli, C Maslach, and T Marek (Eds.). Professional Burnout: Recent Developments in Theory and Research. New York: Francis and Taylor (1993), 135–150.

Cherniss C. Staff Burnout: Job Stress in the Human Services. Newbury Park, CA: Sage Publications (1980).

Chiriboga D, Jenkins G, and Bailey J. Stress and Coping among Hospice Nurses: Test of Analytic Model. Nursing Research (1983), Vol. 32:294–299.

Chiriboga DA and Bailey J. Stress and Burnout among Critical Care and Medical Surgical Nurses: A Comparative Study. Critical Care Nursing Quarterly (1986), Vol. 9:84–92.

Chodron P. When Things Fall Apart. Boston: Shambala (1997).

Christensen J and Suchman A. Introduction. Medical Encounter (2002), Vol. 16:4:2.

Chuck JM, Nesbitt TS, Kwan J, and Kam SM. Is Being a Doctor Still Fun? Western Journal of Medicine (1993), Vol. 159:6:665–671.

Ciarrocchi J. Counseling Problem Gamblers: A Self-Regulation Manual for Individuals and Family Therapy. San Diego: CA: Academic Press (2002).

Clark DC. Prevalence of Psychiatric Risk Factors among First Year Medical Students. Research in Medical Education (1983). Proceedings of the Twenty-Second Annual Conference, Sponsored by the Association of American Medical Colleges.

Clark DC, Eckenfels EJ, Daugherty SR, and Fawcett J. Alcohol-Use Patterns Through Medical School: A Longitudinal Study of One Class. Journal of the American Medical Association (1987), Vol. 257:2921–2926.

Clark DC, Salazar-Grueso E, Grabler P, et al. Predictors of Depression During the First Six Months of Internship. American Journal of Psychiatry (1984), Vol. 141:1095–1098.

Claus K and Bailey J (Eds.), Living with Stress and Promoting Well-being. St. Louis: Mosby (1980).

Clever L. Who Is Sicker: Patients—or Residents? Residents' Distress and the Care of Patients. Annals of Internal Medicine (2002), 136:5:393.

Cobb S. Social Support as a Moderator of Life Stress: Presidential Address. Psychosomatic Medicine (1976), 38:5:300–314.

Cohen S, Kamarck T, and Mermelstein R. A Global Measure of Perceived Stress. Journal of Health and Social Behavior (1983), Vol. 24:385–396.

Cole R. Quoted in Dorothy Day: Portraits by Those Who Knew Her, by R Riegle. Maryknoll, NY: Orbis (2003), 140.

Coles C. Medicine and Stress. Journal of Medical Education (1994), Vol. 28:3–4.

Colford JM and McPhee SJ. The Raveled Sleeve of Care: Managing the Stress of Residency Training. Journal of the American Medical Association (1989), Vol. 261:889–893.

Conley S, Bacharach S, and Bauer S. Organizational Work Environment and Teacher Career Dissatisfaction. Education Administration Quarterly (1988).

Constable J. The Effects of Social Support and the Work Environment Upon Burnout among Nurses (Doctoral Dissertation, University of Iowa, 1983). Dissertation Abstracts International (1984), Vol. 44:3713B.

Coombs RH and Fawzy FI. The Impaired-Physician Syndrome: A Developmental Perspective. In CD Scott and J Hawk (Eds.), Heal Thyself: The Health of Health Care Professionals, 44–55. New York: Brunner Mazel Publishers (1986).

Cooper CL, Rout U, and Faragher B. Mental Health, Job Satisfaction and Job Stress among General Practitioners. British Medical Journal (1989), Vol. 298:366–370.

Cordes CL and Dougherty TW. A Review and an Integration of Research on Job Burnout. Academy of Management Review (1993), Vol. 18:4:621–656.

Corrigan PW, Holmes EP, and Luchins D. Burnout and Collegial Support in State Psychiatric Hospital Staff. Journal of Clinical Psychology (1995), Vol. 51:5:703–710.

Corrigan PW, Holmes EP, Luchins D, Buican B, et al. Staff Burnout in a Psychiatric Hospital: A Cross-lagged Panel Design. Journal of Organizational Behavior (1994), Vol. 15:65–74.

Council on Mental Health. The Sick Physician: Impairment by Psychiatric Disorders, Including Alcoholism and Drug Dependence. Journal of the American Medical Association (1973), Vol. 223:6:684–687.

Cousins N. Internship: Preparation or Hazing? Journal of the American Medical Association (1981), Vol. 245:377.

Dalai Lama. The Path to Tranquility. New York: Penguin (2000).

Dames K. Relationship of Burnout to Personality and Demographic Traits in Nurses (Doctoral Dissertation, City University of New York, 1983). Dissertation Abstracts International (1983), Vol. 44, 622B.

Danto LA. The Prevention and Cure of Physician Burnout. Western Journal of Medicine (2001), Vol. 174:309–310.

Davis-Sacks ML, Jayartne S, and Chess WA. A Comparison of the Effects of Social Support on the Incidence of Burnout. Social Work (1985), Vol. 30:240–244.

Decker FH. Socialization and Interpersonal Environment in Nurses' Affective Reactions to Work. Social Science and Medicine (1985), Vol. 20:499–509.

Delvaux N, Razavi D, and Farvacques C. Cancer Care, a Stress for Health Professionals. Social Science and Medicine (1988), Vol. 27:159–166.

Demerouti E, Bakker AB, Nachreiner F, and Schaufeli WB. A Model of Burnout and Life Satisfaction amongst Nurses. Journal of Advanced Nursing (2000), Vol. 32:2:454–464.

Dewe PJ. Identifying the Causes of Nurses' Stress: A Survey of New Zealand Nurses. Work and Stress (1987), Vol. 7:5–15.

Dickstein LJ. Medical Students and Residents: Issues and Needs. In LS Goldman, M Myers, and LJ Dickstein (Eds.), The Handbook of Physician Health. Chicago: American Medical Association (2000), 161–179.

Dickstein LJ and Elkes J. A Health Awareness Workshop: Enhancing Coping Skills in Medical Students. In CD Scott and J Hawk (Eds.), Heal Thyself: The Health of Health Care Professionals. New York: Brunner Mazel Publishers (1986), 269–281.

Dignam JT, Barrera M Jr, and West SG. Occupational Stress, Social Support, and Burnout Among Correctional Officers. American Journal of Community Psychology (1986), Vol. 14:2:177–193.

Dilts SJ and Gendel MH. Substance Use Disorders. In LS Goldman, M Myers, and LJ Dickstein (Eds.), The Handbook of Physician Health. Chicago: American Medical Association (2000), 118–137.

Dohrenwend BP, Shrout PE, Egri G, et al. Nonspecific Psychological Distress and Other Dimensions of Psychopathology. Archives of General Psychiatry (1980), Vol. 37:1229–1236.

Dolan SL and Renaud S. Individual, Organizational and Social Determinants of Managerial Burnout: A Multivariate Approach. Journal of Social Behavior and Personality (1992), Vol. 7:1:95–110.

Domar A and Dreher H. Self-Nurture: Learning to Care for Yourself as Effectively as You Care for Everyone Else. New York: Penguin (2000).

Donnelly JC. Coping and Development During Internship. In Callan JP (Ed.), The Physician: A Professional Under Stress. Norwalk, CT: Appleton-Century-Crofts (1983), 46–80.

Doyle BB and Cline DW. Approaches to Prevention in Medical Education. In The Impaired Physician. New York: Plenum (1983), 51–67.

Druzin P, Shrier I, Yacowar M, and Rossignol M. Discrimination Against Gay, Lesbian and Bisexual Family Physicians by Patients. Canadian Medical Association Journal (1998), Vol. 158:5:593–598.

Dubois D. Renewal of Prayer. Lumen Vitae (1983), Vol. 38:3:273–274.

Ducker D. Research on Women Physicians with Multiple Roles: A Feminist Perspective. Journal of the American Women's Association (1994), Vol. 49:3:78–84.

Ducker DG. Role Conflict for Women Physicians. In CD Scott and J Hawk (Eds.), Heal Thyself: The Health of Health Care Professionals. New York: Brunner Mazel Publishers (1986), 86–109.

Duckitt J. Social Support, Personality, and the Prediction of Psychological Distress: An Interactionist Approach. Journal of Clinical Psychology (1984), Vol. 40:1199–1205.

Duffy JC. Emotional Issues in the Lives of Physicians. Springfield, IL: Charles C Thomas (1970).

Duffy JC and Litin EM. The Emotional Health of Physicians. Springfield, IL: Charles C Thomas (1967).

Dunning D and Story AL. Depression, Realism, and the Overconfidence Effect: Are the Sadder Wiser When Predicting Future Actions and Events? Journal of Personality and Social Psychology (1991), Vol. 61:521–532.

Duxbury ML, Armstrong GD, Drew DJ, and Henly SJ. Head Nurse Leadership Style with Staff Nurse Burnout and Job Satisfaction in Neonatal Intensive Care Units. Nursing Research (1984), Vol. 33:97–101.

Duxbury ML, Henly GA, and Armstrong GD. Measurement of the Nurse Organizational Climate of Neonatal Intensive Care Units. Nursing Research (1982), Vol. 31:83–88.

Eanes B, Richmond L, and Link J. What Brings You to Life: Awakening Spiritual Essence. Mahwah, NJ: Paulist Press (2001).

Eastburg MC, Williamson M, Gorsuch R, and Ridley C. Social Support, Personality, and Burnout in Nurses. Journal of Applied Social Psychology (1994), Vol. 24:14:1233–1250.

Edelwich J and Brodsky A. Burnout. New York: Human Sciences Press (1980), 14.

Edwards D, Burnard P, Coyle D, Fothergill A, and Hannigan B. Stress and Burnout in Community Mental Health Nursing: A Review of the Literature. Journal of Psychiatric and Mental Health Nursing (2000), Vol. 7:7–15.

Edwards R. "Compassion Fatigue": When Listening Hurts. Washington, DC: American Psychological Association (1995), 34–35.

Eisenberg L and Kleinman A (Eds.), Clinical Social Scientist. In, The Relevance of Social Science for Medicine. Dordrecht: Reidel (1981), 7–20.

Ellard J. The Disease of Being a Doctor. Medical Journal of Australia (1974), Vol. 2:318–323.

Elliott-Binns C, Bingham L, and Perle E. Managing Stress in the Primary Care Team Oxford: Blackwell Scientific Publications (1997).

Ende J. Feedback in Clinical Medical Education. Journal of the American Medical Association (1983), Vol. 250:777–781.

Enders LE and Mercier JM. Treating Chemical Dependency: The Need for Including the Family. International Journal of Addictions (1993), Vol. 28:507–519.

Epstein LC, Thomas CB, Shaffer JW, and Perlin S. Clinical Prediction of Physician Suicide Based on Medical Student Data. The Journal of Nervous and Mental Disease (1973), Vol. 156:19–29.

Ewers P, Bradshaw T, McGovern J, and Ewers B. Does training in psychosocial interventions reduce burnout rates in forensic nurses? Journal of Advanced Nursing (2002), Vol. 37:5:470–476.

Fabri PJ, McDaniel MD, Gaskill HV, Garison RN, et al. Great Expectations: Stress and the Medical Family. Journal of Surgery and Research (1989), Vol. 47:379–382.

Fifth National Conference Set for September 1982. AMA Impaired Physician Newsletter (1981), Vol. 4:3.

Figley C (Ed.). Treating Compassion Fatigue. New York: Brunner-Routledge (2002).

Fimian MJ, Fastenau PS, and Thomas J. Stress in Nursing and Intentions to Leave the Profession. Psychological Reports (1989), Vol. 62:105–111.

Firth H and Britton P. "Burnout," Absence, and Turnover amongst British Nursing Staff. Journal of Occupational Psychology (1989), Vol. 62:55–59.

Firth H, McIntee J, McKeown P, and Britton PG. Maslach Burnout Inventory: Factor Structure and Norms for British Nursing Staff. Psychological Reports (1985), Vol. 57:147–150.

Firth-Cozens J. Predicting Stress in General Practitioners: 10 Year Follow-up Postal Survey. British Medical Journal (1997), Vol. 315:34–35.

Firth-Cozens J. The Psychological Problems of Doctors. In J Firth-Cozens and R Payne (Eds.), Stress in Healthy Professionals: Psychological and Organisational Causes and Interventions. New York: John Wiley and Sons (1999), 79–91.

Firth-Cozens J and Greenhalgh J. Doctors' Perceptions of the Links between Stress and Lowered Clinical Care. Social Science and Medicine (1997), Vol. 44:7:1017–1022.

Firth-Cozens J and Payne R (Eds.), Stress in Health Professionals. New York: Wiley (1999).

Flach F. Putting the Pieces Together Again: A Physician's Guide to Thriving on Stress. New York: Hatherleigh Press (tape).

Foa EB, Steketee G, and Olasov Rothbaum B. Behavioral/Cognitive Conceptualizations of Post-traumatic Stress Disorder. Behavior Therapy (1989), Vol. 20:155–176.

Foner N. The Caregiving Dilemma: Work in an American Nursing Home. Berkeley: University of California Press (1994).

Ford C and Wentz D. Internship: What is stressful? Southern Medical Journal (1986), Vol. 79:595–599.

Ford CV. Emotional Distress in Internship and Residency: A Questionnaire Study. Psychiatric Medicine (1983), Vol. 1:2:143–150.

Forest JM. The Effects of Chronic Exposure to Stresses on the Intensive Care Nurse. (Doctoral Dissertation, California School of Professional Psychology, 1999). Dissertation Abstracts International, AAT.9918487.

Foy DW, Drescher KD, Fitz AG, and Kennedy KR. Post-Traumatic Stress Disorder. In RJ Wicks (Ed.), Clinical Handbook of Pastoral Counseling, Vol. 3. Mahwah, NJ: Paulist Press (2003), 274–288.

Foy DW, Osato S, Houskamp B, and Neumann D. Etiology Factors in Posttraumatic Stress Disorder. In Saigh P (Ed.), Posttraumatic Stress Disorder: A Behavioral Approach to Assessment and Treatment. Oxford: Pergamon Press (in press).

Foy DW, Sipprelle RC, Rueger DB, and Carroll EM. Etiology of Posttraumatic Stress Disorder in Vietnam Veterans: Analysis of Pre-military, Military, and Combat Exposure Influences. Journal of Consulting and Clinical Psychology (1984), Vol. 52:79–87.

Frank E. Self-Care, Prevention, and Health Promotion. In LS Goldman, M Myers, and LJ Dickstein (Eds.), The Handbook of Physician Health. Chicago: American Medical Association (2000).

Franks RD, Getto C, Miller G, and Tardiff K. Symposium: Medical Student and Resident "Impairments": Prediction, Early Recognition, and Intervention. Should They Be Rehabilitated or Should They Be Removed? University of Colorado School of Medicine, 321–328.

Freeborn D. Satisfaction, Commitment and Well-being among HMO Physicians. Permanente Journal (1998), Vol. 2:22–30.

Freid Y, et al. The Physiological Measurement of Work Stress: A Critique. Personnel Psychology (1984), Vol. 37:583–615.

Freudenberger H. Impaired Clinicians: Coping with Burnout. In PA Keller and L Ritt (Eds.), Innovations in Clinical Practice: A Sourcebook, Vol 3. Sarasota, FL: Professional Resource Exchange (1984), 223.

Freudenberger H. Staff Burnout. Journal of Social Issues (1974), Vol. 30:159–165.

Freudenberger H. The Staff Burn-out Syndrome in Alternative Institutions. Psychotherapy: Theory, Research and Practice (1975), Vol. 12:1:73–82.

Freudenberger HJ. The Health Professional in Treatment: Symptoms, Dynamics, and Treatment Issues. In CD Scott and J Hawk (Eds.), Heal Thyself: The Health of Health Care Professionals. New York: Brunner Mazel Publishers (1986), 185–193.

Freudenberger HJ and North G. Women's Burnout: How to Spot It, How to Reverse It, and How to Prevent It. Garden City, NY: Doubleday and Company (1985).

Friedman RC, Bigger JT, and Kornfeld DS. The Intern and Sleep Loss. New England Journal of Medicine (1971), Vol. 285:4:201–203.

Gabbard G and Menninger R. Medical Marriages. Washington, DC: American Psychiatric Press (1988), 35.

Gabbard GO. The Role of Compulsiveness in the Normal Physician. Journal of American Medical Association (1985), Vol. 254:20:2926–2929.

Gaertner K. Work Satisfaction and Family Responsibility Correlates of Employment among Nurses. Work and Occupations (1984), Vol. 11:439–460.

Gallegos KV, Lubin BH, Bowers C, et al. Relapse and Recovery: Five to Ten Year Follow Up Study of Chemically Dependent Physicians—The Georgia Experience. Maryland Medical Journal (1992), Vol. 41:315–319.

Gallegos KV and Norton M. Characterization of Georgia's Impaired Physicians Program Treatment Population: Data and Statistics. Journal of Medical Association of Georgia (1984), Vol. 73:755–758.

Ganster DC. Type A Behavior and Job Stress. In JM Ivancevich and DC Ganster (Eds.), Job Stress: From Theory to Suggestion. New York: Haworth Press (1987).

Garden AM. Depersonalization: A Valid Dimension of Burnout? Human Relations (1987), Vol. 40:9:545–560.

Garfinkel PE and Waring EM. Personality, Interests, and Emotional Disturbance in Psychiatric Residents. American Journal of Psychiatry (1981), Vol. 138:541–551.

Garmezy N and Masten AS. Stress, competence, and resilience: Common frontiers for therapist and psychopathologist. Behavioral Therapy (1986), Vol. 17:500–521.

Gautam M. Depression and Anxiety. In LS Goldman, M Myers, and LJ Dickstein (Eds.), The Handbook of Physician Health. Chicago: American Medical Association (2000), 80–94.

Gay JE. Nursing a Stressful Occupation—Prove It! Journal of Royal Society of Health (1983), Vol. 103:78–81.

Gentry ED and Parkes KR. Psychologic Stress in Intensive Care Units and Nonintensive Care Unit Nurses: A Review of the Past Decade. Heart and Lung (1982), Vol. 4:43–47.

Gerber LA. Married to Their Careers: Career and Family Dilemma in Doctors' Lives. New York: Tavistock (1983).

Geurts S, Rutte C, and Peeters M. Antecedents and Consequences of Work-Home Interference among Medical Residents. Social Science and Medicine (1999), Vol. 48:1135–1148.

Gilbert SP. Ethical Issues in the Treatment of Severe Psychopathology in University and College Counseling Centers. Journal of Counseling and Development (1992), Vol. 70:695–699.

Gill J. Burnout: A Growing Threat in Ministry. Human Development (1980), Vol. 1:2:21, 24–25.

Girard DE, Elliot DL, Hickam DH, Sparr L, Clarke NG, et al. The Internship—A Prospective Investigation of Emotions and Attitudes (1986), Vol. 144:93–98.

Girard DE, Sack RL, Reuler JB, Chang MK, and Nardone DA. Survival of the Medical Internship. Forum Med (1980), Vol. 3:460–463.

Glass DC. Toward a Theory of Occupational Burnout. Unpublished manuscript. State University of New York at Stony Brook (1986).

Glass DC, McKnight JD, and Valdimarsdottir H. Depression, Burnout, and Perceptions of Control in Hospital Nurses. Journal of Consulting and Clinical Psychology (1993), Vol. 61:1:147–155.

Gold Y, Bachelor P, and Michael WB. The Dimensionality of a Modified Form of the Maslach Burnout Inventory for University Students in a Teacher-Training Program. Educational and Psychological Measurement (1989), Vol. 49:549–561.

Goldman L, Myers M, and Dickstein L (Eds.), The Handbook of Physician Health. Chicago: American Medical Association (2000).

Goldman LS. When Physicians Become Ill. In LS Goldman, M Myers, and LJ Dickstein (Eds.), The Handbook of Physician Health. Chicago: American Medical Association (2000), 193–204.

Goldman LS, Myers M, and Dickstein LJ. Evolution of the Physician Health Field. In LS Goldman, M Myers, and LJ Dickstein (Eds.), The Handbook of Physician Health. Chicago: American Medical Association (2000), 1–8.

Goldstein MZ. The Aging Physician. In LS Goldman, M Myers, and LJ Dickstein (Eds.), The Handbook of Physician Health. Chicago: American Medical Association (2000), 180–192.

Golembiewski RT, Munzenrider R, and Carter D. Phases of Progressive Burnout and Their Work Site Covariants: Critical Issues in OD Research and Praxis. The Journal of Applied Behavioral Science (1983), Vol. 19:4:461–481.

Golembiewski RT, Munzenrider RF, and Stevenson JG. Stress in Organizations: Toward a Phase Model of Burnout. New York: Praeger (1986).

Goodwin JM, Goodwin JS, and Kellner R. Psychiatric Symptoms in Disliked Medical Patients. Journal of American Medical Association (1979), Vol. 241:1117–1120.

Gordon MJ. A Prerogatives-Based Model for Assessing and Managing the Resident in Difficulty. Family Medicine (1993), Vol. 25:10:637–645.

Gorky M. Gorky: My Childhood. London: Penguin (1996), 173.

Gortmaker SL, Eckenrode J, and Gore S. Stress and the Utilization of Health Services: A Time Series and Cross-Sectional Analysis. Journal of Health and Social Behavior (1982), Vol. 23:25–38.

Graham J. Job Stress and Satisfaction among Palliative Physicians. Palliative Medicine (1996), Vol. 10:184–194.

Graham JR. Risk to Self, Patients, and Profession. Colorado Medicine (1980), Vol. 77:167–172.

Graham LE, Howard CE, Fine JI, Scherwitz L, and Wycoff SJ. Developing a School of Dentistry Wellness Program at the University of California. In CD Scott and J Hawk (Eds.), Heal Thyself: The Health of Health Care Professionals. New York: Brunner Mazel Publishers (1986), 282–295.

Grant R. Trauma in Missionary Life. Unpublished manuscript (1993), 1–14.

Gravenstein JS, Kory WP, and Marks RG. Drug Abuse by Anesthesia Personnel. Anesthesia and Analgesia (1983), Vol. 62:467–472.

Gray-Toft P and Anderson JG. Organizational Stress in the Hospital: Development of a Model for Diagnosis and Prediction. Health Sciences Research (1985), Vol. 19:753–774.

Gray-Toft P and Anderson JG. The Nursing Stress Scale: Development of an instrument. Journal of Behavioral Assessment (1981a), Vol. 3:11–23.

Gray-Toft P and Anderson JG. Stress among Hospital Nursing Staff: Its Causes and Effects. Social Science and Medicine (1981b), Vol. 15a:639–647.

Green BL, Grace MC, and Gleser GC. Identifying Survivors at Risk: Long-term Impairment Following the Beverly Hills Supper Club Fire. Journal of Consulting and Clinical Psychology (1985), Vol. 53, 5:672–678.

Greenhaus J, Bedeian A, and Mossholder K. Work Experiences, Job Performance, and Feelings of Family Well-being. Journal of Vocational Behavior (1987), Vol. 31:200–215.

Greenhaus J and Beutell N. Sources of Conflict between Work and Family Roles. Academy of Management Review (1985), Vol. 10:76–88.

Greer JG and Wethered CD. Learned Helplessness: A Piece of the Burnout Puzzle. Exceptional Children (1984), Vol. 50:524–530.

Groenwegen PP and Hutten JBF. Workload and Job Satisfaction among General Practitioners: A Review of the Literature. Social Science Medicine (1991), Vol. 10:1111–1119.

Gross EB. Gender Differences in Physicians' Stress. Journal of American Medical Women's Association (1992), Vol. 47:107–114.

Grout JW, Steffen SM, and Biley JT. The Stresses and the Satisfiers of the Intensive Care Unit: A Survey. Critical Care Quarterly (1981), Vol. 3:35–45.

Groves JE. Taking Care of the Hateful Patient. The New England Journal of Medicine (1978), Vol. 298:16:883–887.

Gueritault-Chalvin V, Kalichman SC, Demi A, and Peterson JL. Work-Related Stress and Occupational Burnout in AIDS Caregivers: Test of a Coping Model with Nurses Providing AIDS Care. AIDS Care (2000), Vol. 12:2:149–161.

Gunderson L. Physician Burnout. Annals of Internal Medicine (2001), Vol. 135:2:145–148.

Hadley J, Cantor JC, Willke RJ, Feder J, and Cohen AB. Young Physicians Most and Least Likely to Have Second Thoughts about a Career in Medicine. Academic Medicine (1992), Vol. 67:3:180–190.

Halenar JF. Doctors Don't Have to Burn Out. Medical Economics (1981), Vol. 58:148–161.

Hannigan B, Edwards D, Coyle D, Fothergill A, and Burnard P. Burnout in Community Mental Health Nurses: Findings from the All-Wales Stress Study. Journal of Psychiatric and Mental Health Nursing (2000), Vol. 7:1277.

Hare J and Pratt CC. Burnout: Differences between Professional and Paraprofessional Nursing Staff in Acute Care and Long-Term Care Health Facilities. Journal of Applied Gerontology (1988), Vol. 7:60–72.

Harrington JM. Working Long Hours and Health. British Medical Journal (1994), Vol. 308:6944:1581–1584.

Harrison D and Chick J. Trends of Alcoholism among Male Doctors in Scotland. Addiction (1994), Vol. 89:1613–1617.

Harwood M. The Ordeal. New York Times Magazine. June 3, 1984, pp 38–48, 70–82.

Haslam D (Ed.), Not Another Guide to Stress in General Practice (2nd edition). Oxford: Radcliffe Medical Press, 2000.

Hassenfeld I and Lavigne G. Issues Raised by Troubled Residents' Need for Psychotherapy. Journal of Medical Education (1987), Vol. 62:608–610.

Haug MR and Lavin B. Practitioner or Patient—Who's In Charge? Journal of Health and Social Behavior (1981), Vol. 22:212–229.

Hawk J and Scott CD. A Case of Family Medicine: Sources of Stress in Residents and Physicians in Practice. In CD Scott and J Hawk (Eds.), Heal Thyself: The Health of Health Care Professionals. New York: Brunner Mazel Publishers (1986), 71–85.

Hay G. The Way to Happiness. New York: Simon and Schuster (1967).

Hayter M. Burnout and AIDS Care-Related Factors in HIV Community Clinical Nurse Specialists in the North of England. Journal of Advanced Nursing (1999), Vol. 29:4:984.

Healy C and McKay M. Identifying Sources of Stress and Job Satisfaction in the Nursing Environment. Australian Journal of Advanced Nursing (1999), Vol. 7:2:30–35.

Heim E. Job Stressors and Coping in Health Professions. Psychotherapy and Psychosomatics (1991), Vol. 55:90–99.

Heins M, Clifton R, Simmons J, et al. Expansion of Services for Medical Students. Journal of Medical Education (1980), Vol. 55:428–433.

Hendrie H, Clair DK, Brittain HM, and Fadul PE. A Study of Anxiety/Depressive Symptoms of Medical Students, House Staff and Their Spouses/Partners. Journal of Nervous and Mental Disorders (1990), Vol. 178:204–207.

Herman MW, Veloski JJ, and Hojat M. Validity and Importance of Low Ratings Given Medical Graduates in Noncognitive Areas. Journal of Medical Education (1983), Vol. 58:837–843.

Heschel A. On Prayer. Conservative Judaism (1970), Vol. XXV:1.

Heschel A. The Insecurity of Freedom. New York: Farrar, Straus, and Giroux (1951).

Heyworth J, Whitley TW, Allison EJ Jr, and Revicki DA. Predictors of Work Satisfaction among SHOs during Accident and Emergency Medicine Training. Archives of Emergency Medicine (1993), Vol. 10:279–288.

Hill HE. The Addicted Physician. Research Publications: Association for Research in Nervous and Mental Disease (1968), Vol. 46:321–322.

Hingley P and Cooper CL. Stress and the Nurse Manager. Chichester, UK: Wiley (1986).

Hipwell AE, Tyler PA, and Wilson CM. Sources of Stress and Dissatisfaction among Nurses in Four Hospital Environments. British Journal of Medical Psychology (1989), Vol. 62:71–79.

Hobfoll SE. The Ecology of Stress. New York: Hemisphere Publishing Corporation (1988).

Holland J. A Doctor's Dilemma. London: Free Association Books (1995).

Holland JC and Holland JF. A Neglected Problem: The Stresses of Cancer Care on Physicians (Oncology Rounds). Primary Care Cancer (1985), Vol. 5:16–22.

Hood R, Spilka B, Budsberger B, and Gorsuch R. The Psychology of Religion. New York: Guilford Press (1996).

House J. Work Stress and Social Support. Reading, MA: Addison, Wesley (1981).

Houskamp B and Foy DW. The Assessment of PTSD in Battered Women. Journal of Interpersonal Violence. In press.

Howell J II and Schroeder D. Physician Stress: A Handbook for Coping. Baltimore, MD: University Park Press (1980).

Howell MC. Stop the Treadmill. We Want to Get Off. New Physician (1974), Vol. 27–30.

Howie J and Porter M. Stress and Interventions for Stress in General Practitioners. In J Firth-Cozens and R Payne (Eds.), Stress in Health Professionals: Psychological and Organisational Causes and Interventions. New York: John Wiley and Sons (1999), 163–176.

Hsu K and Brett J. Mediators, Moderators, and Tests for Mediation. Journal of Applied Psychology (1984), Vol. 144:12:1561–1566.

Hughes PH, Brandenburg N, Baldwin DC, et al. Prevalence of Substance Abuse among US Physicians. Journal of the American Medical Association (1992), Vol. 267:2333–2339.

Hughes PH, Conard S, Baldwin DC, Storr CL, and Sheehan DV. Resident Physician Substance Use in the United States. Journal of the American Medical Association (1991), Vol. 265:16:2069–2073.

Humpel N, Caputi P, and Martin C. The Relationship between Emotions and Stress among Mental Health Nurses. Australian and New Zealand Journal of Mental Health Nursing (2001), Vol. 10:55–61.

Humphrey JH. Stress in the Nursing Profession. Springfield, IL: Charles C Thomas (1988).

Hurwitz TA, Beiser M, Nichol H, et al. Impaired Interns and Residents. Canadian Journal of Psychiatry (1987), Vol. 32:165–169.

Hyde GL and Wolf J. Alcohol and Drug Use by Surgery Residents. Journal of the American College of Surgeons (1995), Vol. 181:1–5.

Ivancevich JM and Matteson MT. Nurses and Stress: Time to Examine the Potential Problem. Journal of Nurse Leader Management (1980), Vol. 11:17–22.

Ivancevich JM and Matteson MT. Stress and Work: A Managerial Perspective. Glenview, IL: Scott Foresman (1980).

Iwanicki EF and Schwab RL. A Cross Validation Study of the Maslach Burnout Inventory. Educational and Psychological Measurement (1981), Vol. 41:1167–1174.

Jackson S. Participation in Decision Making as a Strategy for Reducing Job-Related Strain. Journal of Applied Psychology (1983), Vol. 68:3–19.

Jackson S and Maslach C. After-Effects of Job-Related Stress: Families as Victims. Journal of Occupational Behavior (1982), Vol. 3:63–77.

Jackson S and Schuler R. A Meta-Analysis and Conceptual Critique of Research on Role Ambiguity and Role Conflict in Work Settings. Organizational Behavior and Human Decision Processes (1985), Vol. 36:16–78.

Jackson S, Schwab R, and Schuler R. Toward an Understanding of the Burnout Phenomenon. Journal of Applied Psychology (1986), Vol. 71:630–640.

Jacobson SF and McGrath HM (Eds.), Nurses Under Stress. New York: John Wiley and Sons (1983).

Jaffe DT. The Inner Strains of Healing Work: Therapy and Self-Renewal for health Professionals. In CD Scott and J Hawk (Eds.), Heal Thyself: The Health of Health Care Professionals. New York: Brunner Mazel Publishers (1986), 194–205.

Jaffe DT, Goldstein MS, and Wilson J. Physicians in Transition: Crisis and Change in Life and Work. In CD Scott and J Hawk (Eds.), Heal Thyself: The Health of Health Care Professionals. New York: Brunner Mazel Publishers (1986), 134–146.

James L and Brett J. Mediators, Moderators, and Tests for Mediation. Journal of Applied Psychology (1984), Vol. 69:307–321.

Janssen PPM, de Jonge J, and Bakker AB. Specific Determinants of Intrinsic Work Motivation, Burnout and Turnover Intentions: A Study among Nurses. Journal of Advanced Nursing (1999), Vol. 29:1360–1370.

Jensen P. The Role of the Training Institution in the Treatment and Prevention of Resident Impairment. Presented at the Annual Meeting of the Northern California Psychiatric Society, Monterey, CA, April 10–12, 1981.

Jensen PS. Barriers to Working With Impaired Trainees: A Resident's Viewpoint. Psychiatric Quarterly (1983), Vol. 55:4:268–271.

Jensma JL. Kohut's Tragic Man and the Imago Dei: Human Relational Needs in Creation, the Fall, and Redemption. Journal of Psychology and Theology (1993), Vol. 21:4:288–296.

Jex SM, Huges P, Storr C, Conrad S, et al. Relations among Stressors, Strains, and Substance Use among Resident Physicians. The International Journal of the Addictions (1992), Vol. 27:8:979–994.

Jex SM and Spector PE. The Impact of Negative Affectivity on Stressor-Strain Relationships: A Replication and Extension. Work and Stress (1996), Vol. 10:36–45.

Johnson JV and Hall E. Job Strain, Work Place Social Support, and Cardiovascular Disease: A Cross-Sectional Study of a Random Sample of the Swedish Working Population. American Journal of Public Health (1988), Vol. 78:1336–1342.

Johnson JV, Hall E, and Theorell T. Combined Effects of Job Strain and Social Isolation on Cardiovascular Disease Morbidity in a Random Sample of the Swedish Male Working Population. Scandinavian Journal of Work and Environmental Health (1989), Vol. 15:271–279.

Johnson JV, Hall EM, Ford DE, Mead LA, et al. The Psychosocial Work Environment of Physicians: The Impact of Demands and Resources on Job Dissatisfaction and Psychiatric Distress in a Longitudinal Study of Johns Hopkins Medical School Graduates. Journal of Occupational and Environmental Medicine (1995), Vol. 37:9:1151–1159.

166   Bibliography

Johnson WDK. Predisposition to Emotional Distress and Psychiatric Illness amongst Doctor: The Role of Unconscious and Experiential Factors. British Journal of Medical Psychology (1991), Vol. 64:317–329.

Jones A and Butler M. A Role Transition Approach to the Stresses of Organizationally- Induced Family Role Disruptions. Journal of Marriage and the Family (1980), Vol. 42:367–376.

Jones JW, Barge BN, Steffy BD, Fay LM, et al. Stress and Medical Malpractice: Organizational Risk Assessment and Intervention. Journal of Applied Psychology (1988), Vol. 73:727–735.

Justice B, Gold R, and Klein J. Life Events and Burnout. Journal of Psychology (1981), Vol. 108:219–226.

Kabanoff B. Work and Nonwork: A Review of Models, Methods, and Findings. Journal of Sociology (1982), Vol. 64:596–609.

Kahn S. and Saulo M. Healing Yourself: A Nurse's Guide to Self-Care and Renewal. Albany, NY: Delmar (1994).

Kalliath TJ. A Test of the Maslach Burnout Inventory in Three Samples of Healthcare Professionals. Work and Stress (2000), Vol. 14:35–41.

Kaplan A. Meditation and Kabbalah. York Beach, ME: Samuel Weiser (1982), 3.

Karasek RA and Theorell T. Healthy Work: Stress, Productivity, and the Reconstruction of Working Life. New York: Basic Books (1990).

Kardia D, Bierwert C, Cook CE, Miller AT, and Kaplan M. Discussing the Unfathomable: Classroom-Based Responses to Tragedy. Change (2002), Jan/Feb:19–22.

Kash K, Holland J, Breitbart W, Berenson S, et al. Stress and Burnout in Oncology. Oncology (2000), Vol. 14:11:1621–1633.

Kash KM and Holland JC. Reducing Stress in Medical Oncology House Officers: A Preliminary Report of a Prospective Intervention Study. In HC Hendrie and C Lloyd (Eds.), Educating Competent and Humane Physicians. Bloomington: Indiana University Press (1990), pp 183–195.

Kaufmann GM and Beehr TA. Interactions between Job Stressors and Social Support: Some Counterintuitive Results. Journal of Applied Psychology (1986), Vol. 71:522–526.

Keane TM, Fairbank JA, Caddell JM, and Zimering RT. Implosive (Flooding) Therapy Reduces Symptoms of PTSD in Vietnam Combat Veterans. Behavior Therapy (1989), Vol. 20:245–260.

Keane TM, Fairbank JA, Caddell JM, Zimering RT, and Bender ME. A Behavioral Approach to Assessing and Treating Post-traumatic Stress Disorder in Vietnam Veterans. In C Figley (Ed.), Trauma and Its Wake. Bristol, PA: Brunner and Mazel Publishers (1985), 257–294.

Keeve JP. Physicians at Risk: Some Epidemiologic Considerations of Alcoholism, Drug Abuse, and Suicide. Journal of Occupational Medicine (1984), Vol. 26:503–507.

Keller KL and Koenig WJ. Management of Stress and Prevention of Burnout in Emergency Room Physicians. Annals of Emergency Medicine (1989), Vol. 18:42–47.

Kemery E, Mossholder K, and Bedeian A. Role Stress, Physical Symptomology, and Turnover Intentions: A Causal Analysis of Three Alternative Specifications. Journal of Occupational Behaviour (1987), Vol. 8:11–23.

Kilfedder CJ, Power KG, and Wells TJ. Burnout in Psychiatric Nursing. Journal of Advanced Nursing (2001), Vol. 34:383–397.

Kipping CJ. Stress in Mental Health Nursing. International Journal of Nursing Studies (1999), Vol. 37:3:207–218.

Klass P. A Not Entirely Benign Procedure: Four Years as a Medical Student. New York: Putnam (1987).

Koeske GF and Koeske RD. Work Load and Burnout: Can Social Support and Perceived Accomplishment Help? Social Work (1988), 243–248.

Koivula M, Paunonen M, and Laippala P. Burnout among Nursing Staff in Two Finnish Hospitals. Journal of Nursing Management (2000), Vol. 8:149–159.

Kolb LC. A Critical Survey of Hypotheses Regarding Posttraumatic Stress Disorders in Light of Recent Research Findings. Journal of Traumatic Stress (1988), Vol. 1:291–304.

Koocher GP. Adjustment and Coping Strategies among the Caretakers of Cancer Patients. Social Work and Health Care (1979), Vol. 5:145–150.

Koran LM and Litt IF. House Staff Well-being. The Western Journal of Medicine (1988), Vol. 148:97–101.

Korman M, Pate ML, and Chapman TS. Selection of Primary Care as Medical Career: Demographic and Psychological Correlates. Southern Medical Journal (1980), Vol. 73:924–927.

Kornfield J. A Path with Heart. New York: Bantam (1993).

Kosch SG. Physicians, Stress, and Family Life: A Systemic View. In CD Scott and J Hawk (Eds.), Heal Thyself: The Health of Health Care Professionals. New York: Brunner Mazel Publishers (1986), 110–133.

Kottler J. On Being a Therapist. San Francisco: Jossey-Bass (1986), 8.

Kottler J and Hayler R. What You Never Learned in Graduate School: A Survival Guide for Therapists. New York: Norton (1997).

Krakowski AJ. Stress and the Practice of Medicine: Physicians Compared with Lawyers. Psychotherapy and Psychosomatics (1984), Vol. 42:143–151.

Krakowski AJ. Stress and the Practice of Medicine: The Myth and the Reality. Journal of Psychosomatic Research (1982), Vol. 26:91–98.

Kurtz S, Draper J, and Kurtz J. Teaching and Learning Communications Skills in Medicine. Oxford: Radcliffe Medical Press (1998).

Kushnir T, Cohen AH, and Kitai E. Continuing Medical Education and Primary Physicians' Job Stress, Burnout and Dissatisfaction. Medical Education (2000), Vol. 34:430–436.

Kushnir T and Melamed S. The Gulf War and Its Impact on Burnout and Well-being of Working Civilians. Psychological Medicine (1992), Vol. 22:987–995.

Lachman VD. Stress Management: A Manual for Nurses. New York: Grune and Stratton (1983).

Landau C, Hall S, Wartman S, and Macko MB. Stress in Social and Family Relationships During the Medical Residency. Journal of Medical Education (1986), Vol. 61:654–660.

Landsbergis PA. Occupational Stress among Health Care Workers: A Test of the Job Demands-Control Model. Journal of Organizational Behavior (1988), Vol. 9:217–239.

Larsen R. California Model for Treatment of the Impaired Physician. Western Journal of Medicine (1982), Vol. 137:265–268.

Larsen RC. State Medical Societies: Their Perceptions and Handling of Impairment. In CD Scott and J Hawk (Eds.), Heal Thyself: The Health of Health Care Professionals. New York: Brunner Mazel Publishers (1986), 228–234.

Law JK. Starting a Family in Medical School. Journal of American Medical Association (1997), Vol. 277:9:767.

Lazarus RS. Psychological Stress and the Coping Process. New York: McGraw-Hill (1966).

Lazarus RS and Folkman S. Stress, Appraisal, and Coping. New York: Springer (1984).

Lee MC and Chou MC. Job and Life Satisfaction among Remote Physicians in Taiwan. Journal of the Formosan Medical Association (1991), Vol. 90:681–687.

Lee RT and Ashforth BE. A Longitudinal Study of Burnout among Supervisors and Managers: Comparison between Leiter and Maslach (1988) and Golembiewsky et al. (1986) Models. Organizational Behavior and Human Decision Processes (1993), Vol. 34:369–398.

Lee RT and Ashforth BE. On the Meaning of Maslach's Three Dimensions of Burnout. Journal of Applied Psychology (1990), Vol. 75:6:743–747.

Leech K. San Francisco: Harper and Row (1980), 43–44.

Leigh H and Reiser F. The Patient. Plenum Press, New York (1980).

Leiter MP. Coping Patterns as Predictors of Burnout: The Function of Control and Escapist Coping Patterns. Journal of Organizational Behavior (1990), Vol. 11:123–144.

Leiter MP and Maslach C. The Impact of Interpersonal Environment on Burnout and Organizational Commitment. Journal of Organizational Behavior (1988), Vol. 9:297–308.

Lemon SJ, Sienko DG, and Alguire PC. Physicians' Attitudes Toward Mandatory Workplace Urine Drug Testing. Archives of Intern Medicine (1992), Vol. 152:2238–2242.

Lenhart SA and Evans CH. Sexual Harassment and Gender Discrimination: A Primer for Women Physicians. Journal of the American Medical Women's Association (1991), Vol. 46:77–82.

Levitt M and Rubenstein B. Medical School Faculty Attitudes Toward Applicants and Students with Emotional Problems. Journal of Medical Education (1967), Vol. 34:430–436.

Lewis DC. Doctors and Drugs. New England Journal of Medicine (1986), Vol. 315:826–828.

Lewiston NJ, Conley J, and Blessing-Moore J. Measurement of Hypothetical Burnout in Cystic Fibrosis Caregivers. Acta Paediatrica Scandinavia (1981), Vol. 70:935–939.

Lewy R. Alcoholism in Housestaff Physicians: An Occupational Hazard. Journal of Occupational Medicine (1986), Vol. 28:79–81.

Lief HI, Young K, Spruiell V, et al. A Psychodynamic Study of Medical Students and Their Adaptational Problems: Preliminary Report. Journal of Anesthesia (1993), Vol. 35:696–704.

Lin LS, Yager J, Cope D, and Leake B. Health Status, Job Satisfaction, Job Stress, and Life Satisfaction among Academic and Clinical Faculty. Journal of the American Medical Association (1985), Vol. 254:2775–2782.

Lin N. Social Support and Depression: A Panel Study. Social Psychiatry (1984), Vol. 19:83–91.

Lin N, Dean A, and Ensel WM. Social Support, Life Events and Depression. Newbury Park, CA: Sage Publications (1986).

Lingenfelser TH, Kaschels R, Weber A, Zaiser-Kaschels H, et al. Young Hospital Doctors After Night Duty: Their Task-Specific Cognitive Status and Emotional Condition. Medical Education (1994), Vol. 28:566–572.

Linn BS and Zeppa R. Does Surgery Attract Students Who Are More Resistant to Stress? Annals of Surgery (1984), Vol. 200:638–643.

Linn LS and Wilson RM. Factors Related to Communication Style Among Medical House Staff. Medical Care (1980), Vol. 18:1013–1019.

Linn LS, Yager J, Cope D and Leake B. Health Status, Job Satisfaction, Job Stress, and Life Satisfaction among Academic and Clinical Faculty. Journal of the American Medical Association (1985), Vol. 254:2775–2782.

Linville PW. Self-Complexity as a Cognitive Buffer Against Stress-Related Illness and Depression. Journal of Personality and Social Psychology (1987), Vol. 52:663–676.

Linzer M, Konrad TR, Douglas J, et al. Managed Care, Time Pressure and Physician Job Satisfaction. Journal of General Internal Medicine (2000), Vol. 15:441–450.

Linzer M, Visser MRM, Ort FJ, Smets E, et al. Predicting and Preventing Physician Burnout: Results from the United States and the Netherlands. The American Journal of Medicine (2001), Vol. 111:2:170–175.

Loes MW and Scheiber SC. The Impaired Resident. Arizona Medicine (1981), Vol. 38:777–779.

Love L and Beehr T. Social Stressors on the Job: Recommendations for a Broadened Perspective. Group and Organization Studies (1981), Vol. 6:190–220.

Love M, Galinsky E, and Hughs D. Work and Family: Research Findings and Models for Change. ILR Report, Vol. 25:13–20.

Lowes R. Taming the Disruptive Doctor. Medical Economics (1998), Vol. 67–80.

Lubitz RM, Nguyen DD, and Dittus RS. Medical Student Abuse: Must This Be a Risk of Passage? Journal of General Internal Medicine (1995), Vol. 10:91A. Abstract.

Lutsky I, Hopwood M, Abram SE, et al. Psychoactive Substance Abuse among American Anesthesiologists: A 30 Year Retrospective Study. Canadian Journal of Anesthesia (1993), Vol. 40:915–921.

Lutsky I, Hopwood M, Abram SE, et al. The Use of Psychoactive Substances in Three Medical Specialties: Anesthesia, Medicine and Surgery. Canadian Journal of Anesthesia (1994), Vol. 41:561–567.

Lyons JS, Hammer JS, Johnson N, and Silberman N. Unit-Specific Variation in Occupational Stress Across a General Hospital. General Hospital Psychiatry (1987), Vol. 9:435–438.

MacDonald RA and MacDonald BE. Alcoholism in Residency Program Candidates. The Journal of Medical Education, Vol. 57:692–695.

Maddison D. Stress on the Doctor and His Family. Medical Journal of Australia (1974), Vol. 2:315–318.

Makin PJ, Rout U, and Cooper CL. Job Satisfaction and Occupational Stress Among General Practitioners—A Pilot Study. Journal of Royal College of General Practice (1998), Vol. 38:303–306.

Marmar CR, Foy D, Kagan B, and Pynoos RS. An Integrated Approach for Treating Posttraumatic Stress. Review of Psychiatry (1988), 238–272.

Maslach C. Burned-out. Human Behavior (1976), Vol. 5:16–22.

Maslach C. Burnout—The Cost of Caring. New York: Prentice-Hall Press (1982).

Maslach C. Burnout and Alcoholism. In RR Kilburg, PE Nathan, and RW Thoreson (Eds.), Professionals in Distress: Issues, Syndromes and Solutions in Psychology. Washington, DC: American Psychological Association (1986), 53–75.

Maslach C. Burnout: The Cost of Drug Impairment in Random Samples of Physicians and Solutions in Psychology. Washington, DC: American Psychological Association (1986). 53–75.

Maslach C. Job Burnout: How People Cope. Public Welfare (1978), 56–58.

Maslach C. The Client Role in Staff Burn-Out. Journal of Social Issues (1978), Vol. 34:11–124.

Maslach C and Jackson S. Burnout in Organizational Settings. Applied Social Psychology Annual (1984a),Vol. 5:133–153.

Maslach C and Jackson S. Patterns of Burnout among a National Sample of Public Contact Workers. Journal of Health and Human Resources Administration (1984b),Vol. 7:189–212.

Maslach C and Jackson S.The Role of Sex and Family Variables in Burnout. Sex Roles (1985),Vol. 12:7/8:837–851.

Maslach C and Jackson SE. Burned-Out Cops and Their Families. Psychology Today (1979),Vol. 59–62.

Maslach C and Jackson SE. Human Services Survey. Palo Alto, CA: Consulting Psychologists Press (1986).

Maslach C and Jackson SE.The Measurement of Experienced Burnout. Journal of Occupational Behaviour (1981),Vol. 2:99–113.

Maslach C and Pines A. The Burn-Out Syndrome in the Day Care Setting. Child Care Quarterly (1977),Vol. 6:100–113.

Matteson MT and Ivancevich JM. Controlling Work Stress: Effective Human Resource and Management Strategies. 1987, Jossey-Bass Publishers, San Francisco, pp 239–249.

Matthews DA, Classen DC, Williams JL, and Cotton JP. A Program to Help Interns Cope with Stresses in an Internal Medicine Residency. Journal of Medical Education (1988),Vol. 63:539–547.

Matthews DB. A Comparison of Burnout in Selected Occupational Fields.The Career Development Quarterly (1990),Vol. 38:230–239.

Mawardi BH. Satisfactions, Dissatisfactions, and Causes of Stress in Medical Practice. Journal of American Medical Association (1979), Vol. 241:1483–1486.

May HJ, Revicki DA, and Jones JG. Professional Stress and the Practicing Family Physician. South Medical Journal (1983),Vol. 76:1273–1276.

Mazie B. Job Stress, Psychological Health, and Social Support of Family Practice Residents. Journal of Medical Education (1985),Vol. 60:935–941.

McAuliffe WE, Rohman M, Santagelo S, et al. Psychoactive Drug Use among Practicing Physicians and Medical Students. New England Journal of Medicine (1986), 805–810.

McAuliffe WE, Santangelo S, Gringas J, Sobol A, and Magnuson E. Use of Controlled and Uncontrolled Substances by Pharmacists and Pharmacy Students. American Journal of Hospital Pharmacists (1987b),Vol. 44:311–317.

McAuliffe WE, Santangelo S, Magnuson E, Sobol A, et al. Risk Factors of Drug Impairment in Random Samples of Physicians and Medical Students. International Journal of Addictions (1987a),Vol. 22:825–841.

McCaffrey RJ and Fairbank JA. Behavioral Assessment and Treatment of Accident-Related Posttraumatic Stress Disorder: Two Case Studies. Behavior Therapy (1985),Vol. 16:406–416.

McCall TB. The Impact of Long Working Hours on Resident Physicians. New England Journal of Medicine (1988), Vol. 318:775–778.

McCauley J. Give Me Strength: Spirituality in the Medical Encounter. Medical Affairs Department/Johns Hopkins University (tape).

McCauley J (Developed by). "Give Me Strength:" Spirituality in the Medical Encounter Medical Affairs Department/Johns Hopkins University.

McCauley J and Koenig H. Plans to Prosper: A Patient Guide to Faith and Health. Baltimore: Medical Affairs Department/Johns Hopkins University (tape).

McCauley J and Koenig H (Developed by). "Plans to Prosper:" A Patient Guide to Faith and Health Baltimore: Medical Affairs Department/Johns Hopkins University.

McConnel E. Burnout in the Nursing Profession. St. Louis: Mosby (1982).

McCranie E and Brandsma J. Personality Antecedents of Burnout among Middle-Aged Physicians. Behavioral Medicine (1984), Vol. 14:30–35.

McCue JD. Occasional Notes—The Distress of Internship: Causes and Prevention. The New England Journal of Medicine (1985), Vol. 312:449–452.

McCue JD. Special Article—The Effects of Stress on Physicians and Their Medical Practice. The New England Journal of Medicine (1982), Vol. 306:458–463.

McDermott D. Professional Burnout and Its Relation to Job Characteristics, Satisfaction, and Control. Journal of Human Stress (1984), Vol. 10:79–85.

McElroy AM. Burnout—A Review of the Literature with Application to Cancer Nursing. Cancer Nursing (1982), Vol. 5:211–217.

McKnight JD and Glass DC. Perceptions of Control, Burnout, and Depressive Symptomatology: A Replication and Extension. Journal of Consulting and Clinical Psychology (1995), Vol. 63:3:490–494.

McMurray JE, Williams W, Schwartz ME, et al. for the SGIM Career Satisfaction Study Group. Physician Job Satisfaction: Developing a Model Using Qualitative Data. Journal of General Internal Medicine (1997), Vol. 12:711–714.

McNamara RM and Margulies JL. Chemical Dependency in Emergency Medicine Residency Programs: Perspective of the Program Directors. Annals of Emergency Medicine (1994), Vol. 23:5:1072–1076.

Meadow KP. Burnout Professionals Working with Deaf Children. American Annals of the Deaf (1981), Vol. 126:13–22.

Mechanick P, Mintz J, Gallagher J, Lapid G, et al. Nonmedical Drug Use among Medical Students. Archives of General Psychiatry (1973), Vol. 29:48–50.

Mee CL. Battling Burnout. Nursing (2002), Vol. 32:8–ff.

Meek D. The Impaired Physician Program of the Medical Society of the District of Columbia. Maryland Medical Journal (1992), Vol. 41:321–323.

Meier ST. The Construct Validity of Burnout. Journal of Occupational Psychology (1984), Vol. 57:211–219.

Meier ST. Toward a Theory of Burnout. Human Relations (1983), Vol. 36:10:899–910.

Melchior MEW, Philipsen H, Abu-Saad HH, Halfens RJG, van de Berg AA, et al. The Effectiveness of Primary Nursing on Burnout among Psychiatric Nurses in Long-Stay Settings. Journal of Advanced Nursing (1996), Vol. 24:694–703.

Menk EJ, Baungarten RK, Kingsley CP, et al. Success of Reentry into Anesthesiology Training Programs by Residents Who Have a History of Substance Abuse. Journal of American Medical Association (1990), Vol. 263:3060–3062.

Mentink J and Scott CD. Implementing a Self-Care Curriculum. In CD Scott and J Hawk (Eds.), Heal Thyself: The Health of Health Care Professionals. New York: Brunner Mazel Publishers (1986), 235–256.

Merton T. A Vow of Conversation. New York: Farrar, Straus, and Giroux (1988).

Messner E. Resilience Enhancement for the Resident Physician. Devant, OK: Essential Medical Information Systems (1993).

Miller M and Potter R. Professional Burnout among Speech-Language Pathologists. ASHA (1982), Vol. 24:177–180.

Mizrahi T. Managing Medical Mistakes: Ideology, Insularity, and Accountability among Internist-in-Training. Social Science and Medicine (1984), Vol. 19:135–146.

Modlin HC and Montes A. Narcotic Addiction in Physicians. Am Journal of Psychiatry (1964), Vol. 121:358–365.

Morgan LD and Hellkamp DT. Burnout among Consulting Psychologists in Division 13 of APA. Consulting Psychology Bulletin (Summer 1991), 1–6.

Moss F and Paice E. Getting Things Right for the Doctor in Training. In J Firth-Cozens and R Payne (Eds.), Stress in Health Professionals: Psychological and Organisational Causes and Interventions. New York: John Wiley and Sons (1999), 203–218.

Muldasy T. Burnout and Health Professionals: Manifestations and Management. Norwalk, CT: Appleton-Century-Crofts (1983).

Mumford E. Editorial: Stress in the Medical Career. Journal of Medical Education (1983), Vol. 58:436–437.

Murphy LR. Organisational Interventions to Reduce Stress in Health Care Professionals. In J Firth-Cozens and R Payne (Eds.), Stress in Healthy Professionals: Psychological and Organisational Causes and Interventions. New York: John Wiley and Sons (1999), 149–162.

Muscroft J and Hicks C. A Comparison of Psychiatric Nurses' and General Nurses' Reported Stress and Counseling Needs: A Case Study Approach. Journal of Advanced Nursing (1998), Vol. 27:1317–1326.

Myers M. Physicians and Intimate Relationships. In LS Goldman, M Myers, and LJ Dickstein (Eds.), The Handbook of Physician Health. Chicago: American Medical Association (2000), 52–79.

Myers M and Dickstein LJ (Eds.). The Handbook of Physician Health. Chicago: American Medical Association (2000), 9–16.

Myers T and Weiss E. Substance Use by Interns and Residents: An Analysis of Personal, Social and Professional Differences. British Journal of Addict (1987), Vol. 25:34–54, 59.

Nagy S. Burnout and Selected Variables as Components of Occupational Stress. Psychological Reports (1985), Vol. 56:195–200.

Nagy S and Davis LG. Burnout: A Comparative Analysis of Personality and Environmental Variables. Psychological Reports (1985), Vol. 57:1319–1326.

Neiblum DR. The Horror of Diagnosis. Pennsylvania Medicine (1989), Vol. 40–41.

Nesbitt J. The Sick Doctor Statute: A New Approach to an Old Problem. Federal Bulletin (1970), Vol. 57, 266–279.

Neser WB, Thomas J, Semenya K, and Thomas DJ. Type A Behavior and Black Physicians: The Meharry Cohort Study. Journal of the National Medical Association (1988), Vol. 80:7:733–736.

Newton TJ and Keenan A. Role Stress Reexamined: An Investigation of Role Stress Predictors. Organizational Behavior and Human Decision Processes (1987), Vol. 40:346–368.

Notman MT. Physician Temperament, Psychology, and Stress. In LS Goldman, M Myers, and LJ Dickstein (Eds.), The Handbook of Physician Health. Chicago: American Medical Association (2000), 39–51.

Nouwen H. Making All Things New. New York: Harper and Row (1981), 33.

Nouwen H. The Way of the Heart. New York: Seabury/Harper Collins (1981), 20.

Novack DH, Suchman AL, Clark W, Epstein RM, et al. Calibrating the Physician: Personal Awareness and Effective Patient Care. Journal of American Medical Association (1997), Vol. 278:6:502–509.

Numerof RE and Abrams MN. Sources of Stress among Nurses: An Empirical Investigation. Journal of Human Stress (Summer 1984), 88–99.

O'Brien M. Spirituality in Nursing. Sudbury, MA: Jones and Bartlett Publishers (2003).

O'Brien M. Spirituality in Nursing: Standing on Holy Ground (2nd edition). Boston: Jones and Bartlett (2003).

O'Connor PG and Spickard A. Physician Impairment by Substance Abuse. Medical Clinics of North America (1997), Vol. 81:4:1037–1052.

Olkinuora M, Asp S, Juntunen J, Kauttu K, et al. Stress Symptoms, Burnout, and Suicidal Thoughts in Finnish Physicians. Social Psychiatry and Psychiatric Epidemiology (1990), Vol. 25:81–86.

Onady A, Rodenhauser P, and Markert RJ. Effects of Stress and Social Phobia on Medical Students' Specialty Choices. Journal of Medical Education (1988), Vol. 63:162–169.

Orioli EM. Caring for the Health and Wellness of the Healer Within the Health Care Institution. In CD Scott and J Hawk (Eds.), Heal Thyself: The Health of Health Care Professionals. New York: Brunner Mazel Publishers (1986), 257–268.

Osipow SH. Psychological Training in Oncology. European Journal of Cancer (1997), Vol. 33:Suppl 6:515–521.

Oyama ON. Investigating the Influence of Peer-Group Cohesion on Residents' Levels of Stress and Performance at Two Residencies. Academic Medicine (June 1991), 66:371.

Paine WS. The Burnout Syndrome in Context. In JW Jones (Ed.), The Burnout Syndrome. Park Ridge, IL: London House Press (1982), 1–19.

Pargament K. Religious Methods of Coping: Resources for Conservation and Transformation of Significance. In EP Shafranske (Ed.), Religion and the Clinical Practice of Psychology. Washington, DC: American Psychiatric Association (1996).

Pargament K. The Psychology of Religion and Coping. New York: Guilford Press (1997).

Parkes KR. Occupational Stress among Student Nurses: A Natural Experiment. Journal of Applied Psychology (1982), Vol. 67:784–796.

Parkes KR. Stressful Episodes Reported by First-Year Student Nurses: A Descriptive Account. Social Science and Medicine (1985), Vol. 20:945–952.

Payne N. Occupational Stressors and Coping as Determinants of Burnout in Female Hospice Nurses. Journal of Advanced Nursing (2001), Vol. 33:396–406.

Pearson T. Physician Life and Career Health and Development. In LS Goldman, M Myers, and LJ Dickstein (Eds.), The Handbook of Physician Health. Chicago: American Medical Association (2000), 228–249.

Perlman B and Hartman EA. Burnout: Summary and Future Research. Human Relations (1982), Vol. 35:283–305.

Peteet JR, Murray-Ross D, Medeiros C, et al. Job Stress and Satisfaction among the Staff Members at a Cancer Center. Cancer (1989), Vol. 64:975–982.

Pfifferling JH. Coping with Residency Distress. Resident and Staff Physician (1983), Vol. 29:105–111.

Pfifferling JH. Cultural Antecedents Promoting Professional Impairment. In CD Scott and J Hawk (Eds.), Heal Thyself: The Health of Health Care Professionals. New York: Brunner Mazel Publishers (1986), 3–18.

Pfifferling JH. Managing the Unmanageable: The Disruptive Physician. Family Practice Management (1997), Vol. 4:10:76–78, 83, 87–92.

Pfifferling JH. The Problems of Physician Impairment. Connecticut Medicine (1980), Vol. 44:587–591.

Piedmont R. Spiritual Transcendence and the Scientific Study of Spirituality. Journal of Rehabilitation (2001), Vol. 67:4–14.

Piedmont R. Spiritual Transcendence as Predictor of Psychosocial Outcome from an Outpatient Substance Abuse Program. Psychology of Addictive Behaviors. In press.

Piedmont RL. A Longitudinal Analysis of Burnout in the Health Care Setting: The Role of Personal Dispositions. Journal of Personality Assessment (1993), Vol. 61:3:457–473.

Pines A. Burnout: A Current Problem in Pediatrics. Current Problems in Pediatrics (1981), Vol. 11:1–32.

Pines A and Maslach C. Characteristics of Staff Burn-Out in Mental Health Settings. Hospital and Community Psychiatry (1978), Vol. 29:233–237.

Pines A, Kafry D, and Etzion D. Job Stress from a Cross-Cultural Perspective. In K Redi and RA Quilan (Eds.), Burnout in the Helping Professions. Kalamazoo, MI: Western Michigan University (1980).

Pines AM. Who Is to Blame for Helpers' Burnout? Environmental Impact. In CD Scott and J Hawk (Eds.), Heal Thyself: The Health of Health Care Professionals. New York: Brunner Mazel Publishers (1986), 19–43.

Pines AM, Aronson E, and Kafry D. Burnout: From Tedium to Personal Growth. New York: Free Press (1981).

Pitts F Jr, Winokur G, and Stewart MA. Psychiatric Syndromes, Anxiety Symptoms and Responses to Stress in Medical Students. American Journal of Psychiatry (1961), Vol. 118:333–340.

Plante A and Bouchard L. Occupational Stress, Burnout, and Professional Support in Nurses Working with Dying Patients. Omega (Westport) (1995–1996), Vol. 32:2:93–109.

Pleck J, Staines G, and Lang L. Conflicts between Work and Family Life. Monthly Labor Review (1980), Vol. 103:29–32.

Puchalski CM. Spirituality and Health: The Art of Compassionate Medicine. Hospital Physician (March 2001), 30–36.

Pullen D, Lonie CE, Lyle DM, Cam DE, and Doughty MV. Medical Care of Doctors. The Medical Journal of Australia (1995), Vol. 162:481–482.

Purcell JM. A Review of the Literature on Burnout in Nurses: Implications for Prevention and Treatment. Columbia: University of Missouri-Columbia (1995), 59.

Purdy RR, Lemkau JP, Rafferty JP, and Rudisill JR. Resident Physicians in Family Practice: Who's Burned Out and Who Knows? Family Medicine (1987), Vol. 19:203–208.

Rafferty JP, Lemkau JP, Purdy RR, and Rudisill JR. Validity of the Maslach Burnout Inventory for Family Practice Physicians. Journal of Clinical Psychology (1986), Vol. 42:3:488–492.

Ramirez AJ, Graham J, Richards MA, et al. Burnout and Psychiatric Disorder among Cancer Clinicians. British Journal of Cancer (1995), Vol. 71:1263–1269.

Ramirez AJ, Graham J, Richards MA, et al. Mental Health of Hospital Consultants: Effects of Stress and Satisfaction at Work. Lancet (1996),Vol. 347:724–728.

Rando TA (Ed.), Loss and Anticipatory Grief. Lexington, MA: Lexington Books (1986).

Rankin ED, Haut MW, Keefover RW, and Franzen MD. The Establishment of Clinical Cutoffs in Measuring Caregiver Burden in Dementia. The Gerontologist (1994),Vol. 34:6:828–832.

Raquepaw JM and Miller RW. Psychotherapist Burnout: A Componential Analysis. Professional Psychology: Research and Practice (1989), Vol. 20:1:32–36.

Razavi D and Delvaux N. Communication Skills and Psychological Training in Oncology. European Journal of Cancer (1997),Vol. 33:suppl 6:515–521.

Reading EG. Nine Years Experience with Chemically Dependent Physicians: The New Jersey Experience. Maryland Medical Journal (1992),Vol. 41:325–329.

Reinhold B. Toxic Work. New York: Plume (1997).

Remen RN. Recapturing the Soul of Medicine. Western Journal of Medicine (2001),Vol. 174:4–5.

Reuben DB. Depressive Symptoms in Medical House Officers: Effects of Level of Training and Work Rotation. Archives of Internal Medicine (1985),Vol. 145:286–288.

Reuben DB. House Officer Responses to Impaired Physicians. Journal of American Medical Association (1990),Vol. 263:7:958–960.

Reuben DB. Psychological Effects of Residency. Southern Medical Journal (1983),Vol. 76:380–383.

Reuben DB, Novack DH, Wachtel TJ, et al. A Comprehensive Support System for Reducing House Staff Distress. Psychosomatics (1984),Vol. 25:815–820.

Revicki DA, May HJ, and Whitley TW. Reliability and Validity of the Work-Related Strain Inventory among Health Professionals. Behavioral Medicine (1991),Vol. 17:111–120.

Revicki DA, Whitley TW, and Gallery ME. Organizational Characteristics, Perceived Work Stress, and Depression in Emergency Medicine Residents. Behavioral Medicine (1993),Vol. 19:74–81.

Rice R, Nea J, and Hunt R. Drug Use among Resident Doctors. Acta Psychiatrica Scandinavia (1980),Vol. 1:37–64.

Rice VH (Ed.), Handbook of Stress, Coping, and Health: Implications for Nursing Research, Theory, and Practice. Thousand Oaks, CA: Sage Publications (2000).

Richardsen AM and Burke RJ. Occupational Stress and Job Satisfaction among Physicians: Sex Differences. Social Science and Medicine (1991), Vol. 33:1179–1187.

Richmond JA. Occupational Stress, Psychological Vulnerability and Alcohol Related Problems Over Time in Future Physicians. Alcoholism, Clinical and Experimental Research (1992), Vol. 16:166–171.

Rilke R. Letters to a Young Poet. New York: Norton (1954).

Rinpoche S. The Tibetan Book of Living and Dying. New York: Harper Collins (1992).

Rockwell F, Rockwell D, and Core N. Fifty-two Medical Student Suicides. American Journal of Psychiatry (1981), Vol. 138:198–201.

Rodman R. Keeping Hope Alive. New York: Harper and Row (1985).

Roeske NC. Risk Factors: Predictable Hazards of a Health Care Career. In CD Scott and J Hawk (Eds.), Heal Thyself: The Health of Health Care Professionals. New York: Brunner Mazel Publishers (1986), 56–70.

Roeske NC. Stress and the Physician. Psychiatric Annals (1981), Vol. 11:245–258.

Rose KD and Rosow I. Physicians Who Kill Themselves. Archives of General Psychiatry (1973), Vol. 29:800–805.

Rosenthal D, Teague M, Retish P, West J, and Vessell R. The Relationship between Work Environment Attributes and Burnout. Journal of Leisure Research (1983), Vol. 15:2:125–135.

Ross M. Suicide among Physicians. Psychiatric Medicine (1971), Vol. 2:189–198.

Rout U, Cooper CL, and Rout JK. Job Stress among British General Practitioners: Predictors of Job Dissatisfaction and Mental Ill-Health. Stress Medicine (1996), Vol. 12:144–166.

Rout U and Rout J. Stress and the General Practitioner. Dordrecht, the Netherlands: Kluwer (1993).

Rout U and Rout J. Understanding Stress in Doctors' Families. Aldershot, England: Ashgate (2000).

Roy A. Suicide in Doctors. Psychiatric Clinics of North America (1985), Vol. 8:2:377–387.

Russell AT, Pasnau RO, and Taintor ZC. Emotional Problems of Residents in Psychiatry. American Journal of Psychiatry (1975), Vol. 132:263–267.

Russell DW, Altmaier E, and Van Velzen D. Job-Related Stress, Social Support, and Burnout among Classroom Teachers. Journal of Applied Psychology (1987), Vol. 72:2:269–274.

Salinksy J and Sacklin P. What Are You Feeling, Doctor? Oxford: Radcliffe Medical Press (2000).

Sambandan S. Burnout. In D Haslam (Ed.), Not Another Guide to Stress in Practice (2nd edition). Oxford: Radcliffe Medical Press (2002), 23–24.

Samkoff JS and McDermott RW. Recognizing Physician Impairment. Pennsylvania Medicine (1988), Vol. 91:36–38.

Samuel SS, Lawrence JS, Schwartz HJ, Weiss JC, and Seltzer JL. Investigating Stress Levels of Residents: A Pilot Study. Medical Teacher (1991), Vol. 13:89–92.

Sanders L. The Case of Lucy Bending. New York: Putnam (1982), 42.

Sauter SL, Hurrell JJ, Cooper CL, eds. Job Control and Worker Health. New York: John Wiley (1989).

Savicki V and Coole E. The Relationship of Work Environment and Client Contact to Burnout in Mental Health Professionals. Journal of Counseling and Development (1987), Vol. 65:249–252.

Schafer W. Stress, Distress and Growth. Davis, CA: Responsible Action (1978).

Schaufeli W, Maslach C, and Marek T (Eds.). Professional Burnout. Florence, KY: Taylor and Francis (1993).

Schaufeli WB and Van Dierendonck D. The Construct Validity of Two Burnout Measures. Journal of Organizational Behavior (1993), Vol. 14:631–647.

Schmoldt RA, Freeborn DK, and Klevit HD. Physician Burnout: Recommendations for HMO Managers. HMO Practice (1994), Vol. 8:2:58–63.

Schnall P, Pieper C, Schwartz J, et al. The Relationship between "Job Strain," Workplace Diastolic Blood Pressure, and Left Ventricular Mass Index: Results of a Case Study. Journal of American Medical Association (1990), Vol. 263:1929–1935.

Schuler R. An Integrative Transactional Process Model of Stress in Organizations. Journal of Occupational Behavior (1982), Vol. 3:5–19.

Schwartz AJ, Black ER, Goldstein MG, Jozefowica RF, and Emmings FG. Levels and Causes of Stress among Residents. Journal of Medical Education (1987), Vol. 62:744–753.

Schwartz RP, White RK, McDuff DR, et al. Four Years Experience of a Hospital's Impaired Physician Committee. Journal of Addictive Diseases (1995), Vol. 14:13–21.

Scott C and Hawk J (Eds.), Heal Thyself: The Health of Health Care Professionals. New York: Brunner Mazel Publishers (1986).

Scott CD. Health Promotion—A Challenging Approach to Health Care. In CD Scott and J Hawk (Eds.), Heal Thyself: The Health of Health Care Professionals. New York: Brunner Mazel Publishers (1986), 209–220.

Seaward B. Managing Stress in Emergency Medical Services. Sudbury, MA: American Academy of Orthopaedic Surgeons/Jones and Bartlett (2000), 9.

Seligman MEP. Learned Helplessness. In E Levitt, B Rubin, and J Brooks (Eds.), Depression: Concepts, Controversies and Some New Facts. Hillsdale, NJ: Erlbaum (1983), 306–327.

Selye H. Stress without Distress. Philadelphia: JB Lippincott (1974).

Sethi BB and Manchanda R. Drug Use among Resident Doctors. Acta Psychiatrica Scandinavia (1980), Vol. 62:447–455.

Shaffer G. Patterns of Work and Nonwork Satisfaction. Journal of Applied Psychology (1987), Vol. 72:115–124.

Shanafelt T, Bradley K, Wipf J, and Back A. Burnout and Self-Reported Patient Care in an Internal Medicine Residency Program. Annals of Internal Medicine (2002), Vol. 136:5:358–367.

Shapiro J, Prislin MD, Larsen KM, and Lenahan PM. Working with the Resident in Difficulty. Family Medicine (1987), Vol. 19:368–375.

Shellenberger S. Clinical Behavioral Scientists: Consultants and Teachers in Family Practice Residencies. In CD Scott and J Hawk (Eds.), Heal Thyself: The Health of Health Care Professionals. New York: Brunner Mazel Publishers (1986), 161–173.

Shinn M, Rosario M, March H, and Chestnut DE. Coping with Job Stress and Burnout in the Human Services. Journal of Personality and Social Psychology (1984), Vol. 46:864–876.

Shirom A. Burnout in Work Organizations. In C Cooper and I Robertson (Eds.), International Review of Industrial and Organizational Psychology, John Wiley and Sons, London (1989).

Siegel B and Donnelly JC. Enriching Personal and Professional Development: The Experience of a Support Group for Interns. Journal of Medical Education (1978), Vol. 53:908–914.

Silver HK and Glieken AD. Medical Student Abuse: Incidence, Severity, and Significance. Journal of American Medical Association (1990), Vol. 263:527–532.

Silverman MM. Physicians and Suicide. In LS Goldman, M Myers, and LJ Dickstein (Eds.), The Handbook of Physician Health. Chicago: American Medical Association (2000), 95–117.

Simpson LA and Grant L. Sources and Magnitude of Job Stress among Physicians. Journal of Behavioral Medicine (1996), Vol. 14:27–42.

Singh G, Singh R, and Jindal K. Drug Use among Physicians and Medical Students. Indian Journal of Medical Research (1981), Vol. 73:594–602.

Skolnik NS, Smith DR, and Diamond J. Professional Satisfaction and Dissatisfaction of Family Physicians. Journal of Family Practice (1993), Vol. 37:3:257–264.

Slaby AE, Lieb J, and Schwartz AH. Comparative Study of the Psychosocial Correlates of Drug Use among Medical and Law Students. Journal of Medical Education (1972), Vol. 47:717–723.

Small GW. House Officer Stress Syndrome. Psychosomatics (1981), Vol. 22:10:860–869.

Smith JW, William FD, and Witzke DB. Emotional Impairment in Internal Medicine House Staff. Journal of American Medical Association (1986), Vol. 255:9:1155–58.

Smythe E. Surviving Nursing. Los Angeles, CA: Western Schools (1994), 27.

Snibbe JR, Radcliffe T, Weisberger C, Richards M, and Kelly J. Burnout among Primary Care Physicians and Mental Health Professionals in a Managed Health Care Setting. Psychological Reports (1989), Vol. 65:775–780.

Snider M and Svenko D. The Physician Burnout Project. Sacramento-El Dorado Medical Society (January 1997).

Sobecks NW, Justice AC, Hinze S, Chirayath HT, et al. When Doctors Marry Doctors: A Survey Exploring the Professional and Family Lives of Young Physicians. Annals of Internal Medicine (1999), Vol. 130:4:312–319.

Sotile W and Sotile M. The Resilient Physician. Chicago: American Medical Association (2002).

Sotile WM and Sotile MO. The Medical Marriage: Sustaining Healthy Relationships for Physicians and Their Families. Chicago: American Medical Association (2000).

Southgate L. What Are You Feeling, Doctor? In J Salinsky and P Sacklin (Eds.), Oxford: Radcliffe Medical Press (2000), viii.

Spears BW. A Time Management System for Preventing Physician Impairment. Journal of Family Practice (1981), Vol. 13:75–80.

Spector PE. Individual Differences in the Job Stress Process of Health Care Professionals. In J Firth-Cozens and R Payne (Eds.), Stress in Health Professionals: Psychological and Organisational Causes and Interventions. New York: John Wiley and Sons (1999), 33–42.

Spickard A. A Survey of Alcohol and Drug Use in Medical Students. Diseases of the Nervous System (1977), Vol. 41–43.

Spickard A and Billings FT. Alcoholism in a Medical School Faculty. New England Journal of Medicine (1981), Vol. 305:1646–1648.

Spickard WA and Tucker PJ. An Approach to Alcoholism in a University Medical Center Complex. Journal of American Medical Association (1984), Vol. 252:1894–1897.

Steffy B and Jones J. The Impact of Family and Career Planning Variables on the Organizational, Career, and Community Commitment of Professional Women. Journal of Vocational Behavior (1988), Vol. 32:196–212.

Steindler EM. The Role of Professional Organizations in Developing Support. In CD Scott and J Hawk (Eds.), Heal Thyself: The Health of Health Care Professionals. New York: Brunner Mazel Publishers (1986), 221–227.

Steinert Y and Levitt C. Working with the "Problem" Resident: Guidelines for Definition and Intervention. Family Medicine (1993), Vol. 25:10:627–632.

Steinert Y, Magonet G, Rubin G, and Carson K. The Emotional Well-being of Housestaff: A Comparison of Residency Training Programs. Canadian Family Physician (1991), Vol. 37:2130–2138.

Steinmetz J, Blankenship J, Brown L, et al. Managing Stress Before It Manages You. Palo Alto, CA: Bull Publishing Co. (1980).

Steinmetz J, Proctor S, Hall D, Blankenship J, et al. Rx for Stress: A Nurse's Guide. Palo Alto, CA: Bull Publishing Co. (1984).

Stewart BE, Meyerowitz BE, Jackson LE, Yarkin KL, and Harvey JH. Psychological Stress Associated with Outpatient Oncology Nursing. Cancer Nursing (1982), Vol. 5:383–387.

Stewart MJ, Ellerton ML, Hart G, Hirth A, Mann K, and Meagher-Stewart D. Stress and Coping Among Oncology Nurses in High-Stress Medical Settings. Journal of Occupational Health Psychology, Vol. 3:3:227–242.

Storr A. On Solitude. New York: Bantam (1988), 18.

Stout JK and Williams JM. Comparison of Two Measures of Burnout. Psychological Reports (1983), Vol. 53:283–289.

Stout-Wiegand N and Trent RB. Physician Drug Use: Availability of Occupational Stress? International Journal of Addictions (1981), Vol. 16:317–330.

Strahilevitz A, Yunker R, Pichanik AM, Smith L, and Richardson J. Initiating Support Groups for Pediatric House Officers. Clinical Pediatrics (1982), Vol. 21:529–531.

Strand C. The Wooden Bowl. New York: Hyperion (1988), 2–3.

Strax TE, Wainapel SF, and Welner S. Physicians with Physical Disabilities. In LS Goldman, M Myers, and LJ Dickstein (Eds.), The Handbook of Physician Health. Chicago: American Medical Association (2000), 17–38.

Stull DE, Kosloski K and Kercher K. Caregiver Burden and Generic Well-being: Opposite Sides of the Same Coin? The Gerontologist (1994), Vol. 34:1:88–94.

Sullivan P and Burke L. Results from CMA's Huge 1998 Physician Survey Point to a Dispirited Profession. Canadian Medical Association Journal (1998), Vol. 159:5:525–529.

Sullivan PJ. Occupational Stress in Psychiatric Nursing. Journal of Advanced Nursing (1993), Vol. 18:591–601.

Sutherland VJ and Cooper CL. Identifying Distress among General Practitioners: Predictors of Psychological Ill-Health and Job Dissatisfaction. Social Science and Medicine (1993), Vol. 37:575–581.

Sutherland VJ and Cooper CL. Job Stress, Satisfaction and Mental Health among General Practitioners Before and After Introduction of New Contract. British Medical Journal (1992), Vol. 304:1545–1548.

Swanson V, Power K, and Simpson R. A Comparison of Stress and Job Satisfaction in Male and Female GPs and Consultants. Stress Medicine (1996), Vol. 12:17–26.

Taintor Z, Morphy M, and Pearson M. Stress and Growth Factors in Psychiatric Residency Training. Psychiatry Quarterly (1981), Vol. 53:163–169.

Takakuwa K, Rubashkin N, and Herzig K (Eds.), What I Learned in Medical School: Personal Stories of Young Doctors. Berkeley: University of California Press (2004).

Talbott GD. The Impaired Physician and Intervention: A Key to Recovery. Journal of Florida Medical Association (1982), Vol. 69:793–797.

Talbott GD and Benson EB. The Impaired Physician: The Dilemma of Identification. Postgraduate Medicine (1980), Vol. 68:56–64.

Talbott GD and Martin CA. Relapse and Recovery: Special Issues for Chemically Dependent Physicians. Journal of Medical Association of Georgia (1984), Vol. 73:763–769.

Talbott GD and Martin CA. Treating Impaired Physicians: Fourteen Keys to Success. Virginia Medicine (1986), Vol. 113:95–99.

Tate P. The Doctor's Communication Handbook. Oxford: Radcliffe Medical Press (2001).

Taylor SE and Brown JD. Illusion and Well-being: A Social Psychological Perspective on Mental Health. Psychological Bulletin (1988), Vol. 103:193–210.

Tetrick LE and LaRocco JM. Understanding, Prediction, and Control as Moderators of the Relationships between Perceived Stress, Satisfaction, and Psychological Well- Being. Journal of Applied Psychology (1987), Vol. 72:538–543.

Theorell T. The Psycho-Social Environment, Stress, and Coronary Heart Disease. In M Marmot and P Elliott (Eds.), Coronary Heart Disease Epidemiology. Oxford: Oxford University Press (1992), 256–273.

Thomas CB. What Becomes of Medical Students: The Dark Side. Johns Hopkins Medical Journal (1976), Vol. 138:185–195.

Thomas RB, Luber SA, and Smith JA. A Survey of Alcohol and Drug Use in Medical Students. Diseases of the Nervous System (1977), pp. 41–43.

Thomas S. Transforming Nurses' Stress and Anger: Steps Toward Healing. New York: Springer (2004).

Thompson SC and Spacapan S. Perceptions of Control in Vulnerable Populations. Journal of Social Issues (1991), Vol 47:1–22.

Toth EL, Collinson K, Ryder C, Goldsand G, and Jewell LD. Committee to Prevent and Remediate Stress among Housestaff at the University of Alberta. Canadian Medical Association Journal (1994), Vol. 150:1593–1597.

Turner RJ, Frankel BG, and Levin DM. Social Support: Conceptualization, Measurement and Implications for Mental Health. Research in Community Mental Health (1983), Vol. 3:67–111.

Tyler PA, Carroll D, and Cunningham SE. Stress and Well Being in Nurses: A Comparison of the Public and Private Sectors. International Journal of Nursing Studies (1991), Vol. 28:125–130.

Tyson, PD, Pongruengphant R, and Aggarwal B. Coping with Organizational Stress among Hospital Nurses in Southern Ontario. International Journal of Nursing Studies (2002), Vol. 39:4:453–459.

Ullrich A and FitzGerald P. Stress Experienced by Physicians and Nurses in the Cancer Ward. Social Science and Medicine (1990), Vol. 31:9:1013–1022.

Vachon ML, Lyall AL, and Freeman SJJ. Measurement and Management of Stress in Health Professionals Working with Advanced Cancer Patients. Death Education (1978), Vol. 1:365–375.

Vachon MLS. Occupational Stress in the Care of the Critically Ill, the Dying and the Bereaved. Washington, DC: Hemisphere Publishing Corp (1987).

Vaillant GE. Physician, Cherish Thyself: The Hazards of Self Prescribing. Journal of American Medical Association (1992), Vol. 267:17:2373–2374.

Vaillant GE, Sobowale N, and McArthur C. Some Psychological Vulnerabilities of Physicians. The New England Journal of Medicine (1972), Vol. 287:8:372–375.

Valko RJ and Clayton PJ. Depression in the Internship. Diseases of the Nervous System (1975), Vol. 36:26–29.

Van Dierendonck D, Schaufeli WB, and Sixma HJ. Burnout Among General Practitioners: A Perspective From Equity Theory. Journal of Social and Clinical Psychology (1994), Vol. 13:1:86–100.

Van Komen GJ (2000). Troubled or Troubling Physicians: Administrative Responses. In LS Goldman, M Myers, and LJ Dickstein (Eds.), The Handbook of Physician Health, 205–227. Chicago: American Medical Association.

Vanlneveld C. Stress in Residency Training: Symptom Management or Active Treatment. Canadian Medical Association Journal (1994), Vol. 150:1549–1551.

Vanlneveld CHM, Cook DJ, Kane SC, King D, and Math B. Discrimination and Abuse in Internal Medicine Residency. Journal of General Internal Medicine (1996), Vol. 11:401–405.

VanYperen NW, Buunk BP, and Schaufeli WB. Imbalance, Communal Orientation, and the Burnout Syndrome among Nurses. Journal of Applied Social Psychology (1992), Vol. 22:173–189.

Vellekoop-Baldock C. Volunteers in Welfare (1990). Sydney: Allen and Unwin.

Veninga RL and Spradley J. The Work/Stress Connection: How to Cope with Job Burnout. Boston, MA: Little, Brown. (1981).

Violations. In LS Goldman, M Myers, and LJ Dickstein (Eds.), The Handbook of Physician Health, 138–160. Chicago: American Medical Association.

Visintini R and Campanini E. Psychological Stress in Nurses' Relationships with HIV- Infected Patients: The Risk of Burnout Syndrome. AIDS Care (1996), Vol. 87:2:183–195.

Visser MRM, Smets EMA, and de Haes JCJM. On Stress and Satisfaction among Medical Consultants: Precursors and Consequences for Health Complaints and Burnout. Canadian Medical Association Journal. Submitted for publication.

Vredenburgh D and Trinkaus R. An Analysis of Role Stress among Hospital Nurses. Journal of Vocational Behavior (1983), Vol. 23:82–95.

Walfish S. Crisis Telephone Counsellors'View of Clinical Interaction Situations. Community Mental Health Journal (1983),Vol. 119:219–226.

Walsh F. The Concept of Family Resilience: Crisis and Challenge. Family Process (1996),Vol. 35:261–281.

Waring EM. A Preventive Approach to Emotional Illness in Psychiatric Residents. Psychiatry Quarterly (1977),Vol. 49:303–315.

Waring EM. Psychiatric Illness in Physicians: A Review. Comprehensive Psychiatry (1974),Vol. 15:519–530.

Weintraub W. The VIP Syndrome: A Clinical Study in Hospital Psychiatry. The Journal of Nervous and Mental Disease (1964),Vol. 138: 2:181–193.

Welner A, Marten S, Wochnick E, et al. Psychiatric Disorders among Professional Women. Archives of General Psychiatry (1979),Vol. 36:169–173.

Wessells D, et al. (Eds.), Professional Burnout in Medicine and the Helping Professions. New York: Haworth Press, 1989.

Wharton AS. The Affective Consequences of Service Work: Managing Emotions on the Job. Work Occup (1993),Vol. 20:205–232.

What every physician's spouse should know . . . survival tips for resident physician spouses. Chicago: American Medical Association Auxilliary, 1984. Available from: American Medical Association Auxiliary, 535 No. Dearborn St., Chicago, IL 60610.

Whippen DA and Canellos GP. Burnout Syndrome in the Practice of Oncology: Results of a Random Survey of 1,000 Oncologists. Journal of Clinical Oncology (1991),Vol. 9:1916–1920.

White RK, Schwartz RP, McDuff DR, et al. Hospital-based Professional Assistance Committees: Literature Review and Guidelines. Maryland Medical Journal (1992),Vol. 41:305–309.

Whitley T and Allison E Jr. Factors Associated with Stress among Emergency Medicine Residents. Annals of Emergency Medicine (1989),Vol. 11:1157–1161.

Whittington R. Attitudes Toward Patient Aggression Amongst Mental Health Nurses in the 'Zero Tolerance' Era: Associations with Burnout and Length of Experience. Journal of Clinical Nursing (2002),Vol. 11:819–825.

Wicks R. After 50: Spiritually Embracing Your Own Wisdom Years. Mahwah, NJ: Paulist Press (1997).

Wicks R. Availability. New York: Crossroad (1986).

Wicks R. Countertransference and Burnout in Pastoral Counseling in Clinical Handbook of Pastoral Counseling, Vol 3. In R Wicks, R Parsons, and D Capps (Eds.), Mahwah, NJ: Paulist Press (2003), 336.

Wicks R. Living a Gentle, Passionate Life. Mahwah, NJ: Paulist Press (1998).

Wicks R. Living Simply in an Anxious World. Mahway, NJ: Paulist Press (1988).

Wicks R. Riding the Dragon. Notre Dame, IN: Sorin Books (2002), 54–46, 109.

Wicks R. Seeds of Sensitivity: Deepening Your Spiritual Life. Notre Dame, IN: AMP (1995).

Wicks R. Simple Changes: Quietly Overcoming Barriers to Personal and Professional Growth. Allen, TX: Thomas More Publishing (2000).

Wicks R. The Stress of Spiritual Ministry: Practical Suggestions on Avoiding Unnecessary Distress. In R Wicks (Ed.), Handbook of Spirituality for Ministers, Vol. 1. Mahwah, NJ: Paulist Press (1995), 254–255.

Wicks R. Touching the Holy: Ordinariness, Self-Esteem, and Friendship. Notre Dame, IN: Ave Maria Press (1992).

Wicks R. Living a Gentle, Passionate Life. Mahwah, NJ: Paulist Press (1998).

Wicks R. Riding the Dragon: 10 Lessons for Inner Strength in Challenging Times. Notre Dame, IN: Sorin Books (2003).

Wicks R and Hamma R. Circle of Friends. Notre Dame, IN: AMP (1996).

Wicks R, Parsons R, and Capps D. Clinical Handbook of Pastoral Counseling, Vol. 3. Mahwah, NJ: Paulist Press (2003).

Wilkinson RT, Tyler PD, and Varey CA. Duty Hours of Young Hospital Doctors: Effects on the Quality of Work. Journal of Occupational Psychology (1975), Vol. 48:219–229.

Williams E, Konrad T, Scheckler W, Pathman D, et al. Understanding Physicians' Intentions to Withdraw from Practice: The Role of Job Satisfaction, Job Stress, and Mental and Physical Health. Health Care Management Review (2001), Vol. 26:1:15.

Williams ES, Konrad TR, Linzer M, et al. Physician, Practice, and Patient Characteristics Related to Primary Care Physician Physical, and Mental Health: Results from Physician Worklife Study. Health Services Research (2002), Vol. 37:121–143.

Williams ES, Konrad TR, Linzer M, et al. Refining the Measurement of Physician Job Satisfaction: Results from the Physician Worklife Study. Medical Care (1999), Vol. 37:1140–1154.

Williams ES, Konrad TR, Linzer M, et al. Understanding Physicians' Intentions to Withdraw from Practice: The Role of Job Satisfaction, Job Stress, Mental and Physical Health. Health Care Management Review (2001), Vol. 26:9–21.

Wilters JH. Stress, Burnout and Physician Productivity. Medical Group Management Journal (May/June 1998), 32–37.

Winefield HR and Anstey TJ. Job Stress in General Practice: Practitioner Age, Sex and Attitudes as Predictors. Family Practice (1991), Vol. 8:140–144.

Wolfe G. Burnout of Therapists. Physical Therapy (1981), Vol. 61:1046–1050.

Yam BMC and Shiu ATY. Perceived Stress and Sense of Coherence among Critical Care Nurses in Hong Kong: A Pilot Study. Journal of Clinical Nursing (2003), Vol. 12:144–147.

Yao DC and Wright SM. National Survey of Internal Medicine Residency Program Directors Regarding Problem Residents. Journal of American Medical Association (2000), Vol. 284:9:1099–1104.

Yasko JM. Variables Which Predict Burnout Experienced by Oncology Nurse Specialists. Cancer Nursing (1983), Vol. 6:109–116.

Yassi A. Assault and Abuse of Health Care Workers in a Large Teaching Hospital. Canadian Medical Association Journal (1994), Vol. 151:1273–1279.

Zaslove M. American Academy of Family Physicians. Curbside Consultation: A Case of Physician Burnout. American Family Physician (2001). http://www.aafp.org/afp/20010801/curbside.html

Zaslove M. The Successful Physician: A Productivity Handbook for Practitioners Gaithersburg, MD: Aspen (1998).

Ziegler JL and Kanas N. Coping with Stress During Internship. In CD Scott and J Hawk (Eds.), Heal Thyself: The Health of Health Care Professionals. New York: Brunner Mazel Publishers (1986), 174–184.

Ziegler JL, Kanas N, Strul WM, and Bennet NE. A Stress Discussion Group for Medical Interns. Journal of Medical Education (1984), Vol. 59:205–207.

Ziegler JL, Strull WM, Larsen RC, et al. Stress and Medical Training. Western Journal of Medicine (1985), Vol. 142:814–819.

Zun L, Kobernick M, and Howes D. Emergency Physician Stress and Morbidity. American Journal of Emergency Medicine (1987), Vol. 6:370–374.

Index